African-American Perspectives on Biomedical Ethics

D0864294

EDITED BY
Harley E. Flack and Edmu~

WITH EDITORIAL ASSISTANCE BY
Dennis McManus

Report of a conference funded by the
Kaiser Family Foundation

GEORGETOWN UNIVERSITY PRESS

Georgetown University Press, Washington, D.C.   20057–1079

Copyright © 1992 by Georgetown University Press. All rights reserved.

Printed in the United States of America
THIS VOLUME IS PRINTED ON ACID-FREE OFFSET BOOK PAPER.

10 9 8 7 6 5 4 3 2 1

Library of Congress Cataloging-in-Publication Data

African-American perspectives on biomedical ethics / [edited by]
    Harley E. Flack, Edmund D. Pellegrino.
            p.   cm.
        1. Medical ethics.   2. Afro-American philosophy.   I. Flack,
    Harley.   II. Pellegrino, Edmund D., 1920-   .
ISBN 0-87840-532-1 (pbk.)
R724.A32   1992   174'.2'08996073--dc20   92-17638

Contents

Edmund D. Pellegrino
Foreword: The Problems and Necessity of Transcultural Dialogue   vii

Harley E. Flack
Introduction: The Confluence of Culture and Bioethics   xiii

Herman Branson
Keynote Address: Africa, African-Americans, and the Origin of a Universal Ethic   1

Jorge L. A. Garcia
African-American Perspectives, Cultural Relativism and Normative Issues: Some Conceptual Questions   11

Tom L. Beauchamp
Response to Jorge Garcia   67

William A. Banner
Response to Jorge Garcia   74

Kwasi Wiredu
The Moral Foundations of African-American Culture   80

Robert M. Veatch
Response to Kwasi Wiredu   94

Marian Gray Secundy
Response to Kwasi Wiredu   99

Kwasi Wiredu
The African Concept of Personhood   104

Laurence Thomas
The Morally Beautiful   118

J. Bryan Hehir
Response to Kwasi Wiredu and Laurence Thomas   127

Leonard Harris
Autonomy Under Duress   133

Edmund D. Pellegrino
Response to Leonard Harris   150

Lynn M. Peterson
Response to Leonard Harris   159

OTHER PAPERS INCLUDED:

Cheryl J. Sanders
Problems and Limitations of an African-American Perspective in Biomedical Ethics: A Theological View   165

James E. Bowman
The Plight of Poor African-Americans: Public Policy on Sickle Hemoglobins and AIDS   173

William A. Banner
Is There an African-American Perspective on Biomedical Ethics?   188

Annette Dula
Yes, There Are African-American Perspectives on Bioethics   193

The Problems and Necessity of Transcultural Dialogue

Contemporary biomedical ethics faces a serious conceptual and practical dilemma. Its origins, modes of reasoning, and moral norms are largely grounded in European and Anglo-American culture. Yet, increasingly, those whom it affects have their moral roots in non-Western cultures. Can Western and non-Western moral values be intermingled without bilateral loss of cultural integrity to both? Are the only alternatives ethical relativism, which is self-destructive, or ethical absolutism, which is morally indefensible? Or is a moral middle ground other than procedural ethics possible?

As a multitude of cultures interact with each other and respond to ethical challenges worldwide, these questions become more urgent. They are particularly acute in the United States, an increasingly culturally polyglot nation. Here Native Americans, African-Americans, Latinos, Asians, and Arabs are in close contact with each other and with the dominant value system. These groups question or reject significant parts of the amalgam of Greek philosophy, Jewish and Christian teachings, and secular humanism, which comprises the dominant ethical system. As these groups grow in political power, they are challenging, changing, and enriching our national mores.

These dilemmas are particularly apparent in the case of Americans of African origin. Their influence on American culture is already evident in a multitude of ways. African-Americans are more aware, better informed, and prouder than ever of the richness and diversity of their African cultural roots. Their value systems are sometimes congruent with, sometimes at odds with, Western European cultural values. There is, as a result, a growing concern that in decisions affecting them, justice is not, or may not be done, to their values and moral norms. This is a genuine concern in biomedical ethics which makes decisions daily about life, death, suffering, procreation, and the uses of professional power.

A serious dialogue between African, African-American, and Western perspectives in biomedical ethics is in order. It can serve as a paradigm of the dialogues that must occur with the other cultures in American society—with Native American, Latinos, Asians, and Arabs. In this volume African-American philosophers examine the conjunction of African and African-American culture with Anglo-American biomedical ethics. They do so in their own way, mindful of the historical realities of black people in America—their enslavement, the injustices and discrimination they have suffered, the stereotyping of their language and culture, and their disadvantaged economic, political, educational, and health status. These philosophers speak in their own voices with the nuances of their own culture enriching their academic prose.

Many moral philosophers trained in the Anglo-American or Eurocentric modes of doing philosophy may find here a disturbing voice. Some will have difficulty accepting some of the papers as "proper" philosophy. Some will misinterpret them as lacking rigor or analytical bite, or as being too anecdotal. Others will miss the usual deference to prima facie principle or to standard ethical theories. But these responses simply underscore the major lesson of this conference, i.e., that to understand another cultural perspective we must listen to that perspective as it is presented, not as we would present it, or as we would want others to present it.

Among these papers are some that fit the "Western" philosophical mold; others rely more heavily on story, metaphorical language, irony, satire, or confrontation. Many African-Americans, though certainly not all, do have a different perspective on ethics than their Western counterparts. They give different weight to certain values or place them in different orders of priority. But their reflections are not, by these differences, made less creditable conceptually or logically.

Those of us educated in the dominant modes of ethical reasoning must listen to hear and to learn. Were all the contributors to this volume to satisfy the criteria of "proper" philosophizing as defined in the Western model, they would fail in their mission. Their diversity of style and methodology illustrates what the conference is about—an authentic perspective on how Africans and African-Americans view the right and the good, the way ethics is linked to their cultural heritage and special experience, and to the experience of their forebears who were black people in a white world. As we read, we must recall Franz Boas's admonition:

It is somewhat difficult for us to recognize that the value we attribute to our own civilization is due to the fact that we participate in this civilization, and that it has been controlling all our actions since the time of our birth.[1]

To recognize how strongly our cultural milieu colors our ethical reflection does not necessitate acceptance of either cultural relativism or absolutism. Anthropologists are especially susceptible to the former; nationalistic ideologues, to the latter. Libertarians abandon substantive for merely procedural ethics.[2] None of these extremes is logically defensible.

Rather, familiarity with our own cultural biases should force us to examine our own ethical presuppositions more critically and to seek more carefully for what other moral systems can contribute, sensitive to what we have in common as human beings and to what divides us. By attempting honestly to comprehend other cultures, we enrich our understanding of our own and purify it of its biases. Only if we do not comprehend culturally who we are, will we be threatened by dialogue with others. In any case, secure or not, to live in America is to engage in transcultural dialogue.

These papers illustrate the diversity of moral perspective and ways of doing ethics even among African-Americans. Some of the authors in this volume, such as William Banner, take a classical "Western" view and maintain that there is no such thing as an African or African-American ethics apart from ethics per se. Others, like Jorge Garcia, use the analytic methodology of "Western" ethical reasoning, but enrich it with the special experience of living as a black person in America. Still others, such as Larry Thomas and Leonard Harris, use a different "voice" to express their concepts; their language draws more strongly on the "story," conceptual cadences, linguistic rhythms, and feelings of African and African-American peoples. Finally, a native African, Professor Kwasi Wiredu, bases his ethical perspective on the idea of humanity that he finds in the Akans of Ghana.

Thus, there is no one African-American perspective, but several different perspectives, each of which may influence daily ethical decisions at the bedside and in public policy. This variety reflects the rich variety of African-American culture. That culture encompasses a wide spectrum of peoples, languages, ethnic strains, and value systems. The temptation is strong to prefer the viewpoints that more closely correspond to what we conceive ethics properly to be and to reject the others. But to do so is to miss the central purpose of this conference—to hear from African-Americans, in their own way of expressing it, their perceptions of ethics and biomedical ethics.

We should not expect these philosophers to be philosophers in the Anglo-American mode who just happen to be African-American. Some do fit this category. Others are African-Americans who also happen to be philosophers, that is, people who reflect critically on their experiences, their own culture, and the world in which it is embedded. It is the same with Catholic, Jewish, or Irish writers. Some are writers who are incidentally Catholic, Jewish, or Irish; others are Catholics, Jews, or Irish women or men who also happen to be able to communicate their experience of living through their writing.

To hear what is being said, the reader must temporarily bracket his or her own cultural presuppositions about what constitutes moral philosophy. This is not to forestall critical evaluation of these ideas but to prevent their preemptory and premature rejection. This would be fatal to any transcultural dialogue and an indefensible position, given the de facto nature of cultural diversity in America.

Equally destructive of dialogue is too ready an acceptance, too facile a judgment on the congruity of African-American with Eurocentric moral philosophy. Certainly, there are moral precepts common to ethical systems in different cultures. But we can arrive at those precepts only after we have made an effort to listen to and to hear one another. Given the history of racial tension in our country, this process is a long way from maturity. Extremists on both sides despair of, or reject, the possibility. Perhaps most destructive of all is the condescending reader, assured by unassailable moral superiority, who listens patiently but hears nothing.

Despite the inherent difficulties, a serious dialogue is essential. There is no way, after all, either globally or in America in particular that cultures can isolate themselves. Transcultural dialogue is a de facto necessity, especially in the matter of biomedical ethics in which so many vexing moral choices are unavoidable.

The necessity for dialogue obtains with other ethnic and cultural groups: Latino, Asian, Arab, Native American, and others for whom the dominant mode of moral philosophy is neither Eurocentric nor Anglo-American. The same sort of problem exists on an even wider scale on the international scene.[3]

The intersection between African-American culture and biomedical ethics depicted in this volume is paradigmatic of the many cultural intersections in our country. We hope in subsequent conferences to examine Native American, Latino, Asian, and Arab perspectives. These dialogues should begin to define the typography of cultural and moral value perspectives that biomedical ethics must take into account if it is to provide a just system of moral guidelines for a pluralistic society.

These perspectives are important to the health of the biomedical ethical enterprise itself. Biomedical ethics in its present form is still a new discipline. It cannot confine itself to one cultural perspective—at least not when the dilemmas it examines are worldwide. The possibility of hermetically sealing one's value system from all others is simply not possible in a world constantly contracted by modern communications technologies.

Transcultural dialogue is a necessity, even a moral requirement for any biomedical ethical enterprise committed to justice in its encounter with peoples of differing cultural values. In this effort, the dialogue between African-American and Western biomedical ethics is a first step. Perhaps in this new field of dialogue, America, the birthplace of biomedical ethics, can also be the birthplace of transcultural dialogue. Biomedical ethics must have this dialogue to serve our multicultural world with justice and sensitivity.

EDMUND D. PELLEGRINO

NOTES

1. Franz Boas, "The History of Anthropology," *Science* 20 (1904): 513-524 as cited in Elvin Hatch, *Culture and Morality* (New York: Columbia University Press, 1983), 39.

2. H. T. Engelhardt, Jr., *Bioethics of Secular Humanism: The Search for a Common Morality* (Philadelphia: Trinity Press International, 1991).

3. E. D. Pellegrino and Patricia Mazzarella, *Transcultural Dimensions of Medical Ethics, A World View*, in press.

INTRODUCTION:

The Confluence of Culture and Bioethics

The importance of recognizing, understanding, and commingling multiple cultures has been, and will continue to be, one of the world's greatest challenges. Whether it be between the black and white races of South Africa, the Arabs and Jews of the Middle East, the Armenians and Slavs of Eastern Europe and the Soviet Union, the Japanese, Chinese and Koreans of Asia, the Indians and the Latinos of South America, or the Native-African-Hispanic-Asian-and European-Americans of the United States, finding the keys to better multicultural relationships is an imperative for global survival.

Superimposed on the multicultural fabric of the world, dramatic medical progress has been made, characterized by the emergence of biomedical ethics. The importance of biomedical ethics as a worldwide phenomena is stated by Edmund Pellegrino.[1] He indicates that the explosion of interest in biomedical ethics over the past two decades is unprecedented in human history. From its beginnings in the United States, biomedical ethics has spread to virtually every industrially and technologically advanced country. Even countries in which biomedical technology is not advanced are experiencing challenges to their traditional values and ways of thinking. So overwhelmed are many of the world's civilizations that attempts to adopt technological and biomedical changes are all but impossible. Instead of sharing in the benefits of technology, e.g., in Africa, South America, or parts of Asia, these countries find their traditional values being torn asunder by changes instigated by colonial-minded wealth seekers and exploitative technology.[2]

The derivations of biomedical ethics are, to date, rooted in western traditions emanating from Greek and Western European traditions. And yet, the Nigerians have a proverb: "Wherever something stands, something else will stand beside it." This means, according to the Nigerian novelist Chinua Achebe, that there is no single way to do anything, nor is there an "absolute" anything.[3]

It is within the context of this proverb that the quest to identify and articulate African-American perspectives on biomedical ethics was begun. Since culture in the United States is neither monolithic nor of a "melting pot nature," the challenge of the African-American perspective on biomedical ethics has been to identify the cultural derivations and nuances that make up a segment of the salad bowl of American peoples in order to enhance the viability (health and health care) of our pluralistic society. Papers contained in this volume represent a comma, punctuating a response to two major questions. First, "Are there African-American perspectives on biomedical ethics?" and second, "If there are, how are they expressed or articulated?"

Before proceeding with an account of the historical development of the project, the editors hasten to point out that numerous ethnic and cultural perspectives (e.g., African-American, Asian-American, Hispanic-American, and Native-American) could and should be articulated on biomedical ethics. The African-American perspective is, however, the only focus of this project. This single focus was selected to develop more thoroughly the philosophical perspective regarded as the quintessential and deterministic starting point for examining the practical issues deriving from (a) a multicultural perspective, or (b) an expanded humanistic perspective on biomedical ethics. The editors strongly recommend and encourage the development of other cultural and ethnic perspectives on biomedical ethics or their admixture into an expanded notion of the humanistic perspective. It is our belief that the model that has been employed for this project is an effective one that can be duplicated to articulate other cultural and ethnic perspectives.

HISTORICAL DEVELOPMENT OF THE PROJECT

The roots of the project reach back to the civil rights movement that swept America in the 1960s and to the search for black identity that rose from the ashes of burning American cities such as Cleveland, Detroit, Washington, D.C., Los Angeles, and Buffalo. The emergence of black pride, black studies programs in higher education, and a preoccupation with black identity were phenomena that touched almost every aspect of human endeavor in the United States. Publications such as *Black Rage* clarioned the disabling effects of racism on a society that had successfully denied Negro Americans the opportunity to find an identity and sense of worth and a chance to relate to others as creators as well as consumers of culture and ideas. In the case of biomedical ethics, this movement is just beginning to blossom two decades later.

As a prelude to the African-American Perspectives on Biomedical Ethics Project, Harley Flack began to articulate some observations on death and dying issues as he worked with African-American and Caucasian patients and their families.[4] He noted the appearance of some perceptible differences in the cognitive, emotive, and spiritual responses of his patients and their families to the approach of death. Consequently, the idea emerged to convene a conference entitled "African-American Perspectives on Death and Dying."

A national conference was planned for 1984. Outstanding speakers were identified, invited, and accepted invitations to participate. The response from the community was so minimal, however, that the conference on death and dying was canceled. Two years later, the notion of broadening "Black Perspectives on Death and Dying" to biomedical ethics was introduced and advanced. In 1987, Harley Flack, then Dean of the College of Allied Health Sciences at Howard University, Dr. Edmund D. Pellegrino, then Director of the Georgetown University Kennedy Institute of Ethics, and Marian Secundy, Professor of Community Health and Family Practice at Howard University, organized and convened a "Think Tank on Black Perspectives on Death and Dying," with support from the Kaiser Family Foundation. The goals of the Think Tank were as follows: (1) to explore strategies for increasing African-American scholarly activity in the field of biomedical ethics, and (2) to recommend a course for continuing a national dialogue on biomedical ethics from an African-American perspective. The discussions and outcomes of the Think Tank are documented in unpublished proceedings.[5]

Two important observations issued from the Think Tank: (1) there was consensus among its participants concerning the existence of an African-American perspective on biomedical ethics, having philosophical and cultural roots that should be explored; and (2) select members of the Think Tank should become the nucleus of a study group for pursuing scholarship in African-American perspectives on biomedical ethics.

It should be noted that the existence of an African-American perspective in biomedical ethics was more a question for the Think Tank than a definitive position. It should also be noted that shortly after its 1987 meeting, a decision was made to use the terminology, "African-American Perspectives" rather than "Black Perspectives." African-American denotes the cultural context of the ideas and issues to be explored. In contrast, black is a color; hence, African-American perspective is the terminology of choice. The papers in this volume have been edited insofar as possible to reflect this choice.

In order to continue the study group's work, a steering committee was organized to chart the course of action for further development of the African-American Perspectives on Biomedical Ethics Project. A steering committee was established with Harley E. Flack and Edmund D. Pellegrino as co-chairs. Other members included Marian Secundy, Ph.D.; Robert Murray, M.D., Professor of Medical Genetics, College of Medicine, Howard University, Washington, D.C.; Mitchell Spellman, M.D., Associate Dean of Clinical Affairs, Harvard University, Cambridge, Massachusetts; and Lynn Peterson, M.D., Director, Medical Ethics, Harvard University, Cambridge, Massachusetts.

THE 1989 CONFERENCE

The next major step in the quest to develop the African-American Perspectives on Biomedical Ethics Project was to convene a conference in 1989 with support from the Brach Foundation. This conference focused on the development of African-American perspectives from philosophical, historical, theological, social, anthropological, and public policy points of view. Papers were prepared and delivered by nationally recognized scholars. Two papers warrant special mention here. The first is by William Banner, Professor Emeritus of Philosophy, Howard University; the second, by Dr. Cheryl Sanders, Professor of Christian Ethics, School of Divinity, Howard University.

In "Is There an African-American Perspective on Biomedical Ethics?", Dr. Banner asserts that the conduct of the sciences of medicine and ethics is incompatible with anything called an "ethnic perspective." He substantiates his position using the Aristotelian logic of definition and classification integrated with Buffon's 1749 thesis regarding uniformity among the human species. Banner concludes with a caution against *the error of redundancy* as pointed out by Aristotle.[6] This redundancy involves "treating as discrete and isolated matters that fall under the same notion," and in this case, according to Dr. Banner, African-American and Western-European perspectives fall under the same notion: both are elements of *a humane perspective.*

Needless to say, Banner's address rekindled the question in the minds of the steering committee, compelling it to renew its examination of the existence of African-American or other "ethnic" perspectives on biomedical ethics.

Cheryl J. Sanders, in "Problems and Limitations of an African-American Perspective in Biomedical Ethics—A Theological View," takes the position that an African-American ethos exists as does a Western-European one within the same moral universe, and "that each brings a valid critique to bear on the other." She hypothesizes a list of seven features in which the ethos or lifestyle of African-Americans and Western-Europeans, respectively, can be contrasted. These contrasts include: (1) the holistic vs. the dualistic; (2) the inclusive vs. the secular; (3) the communalistic vs. the individualistic; (4) the spiritual vs. the secular; (5) the theistic vs. the agnostic or the atheistic, (6) the improvisational vs. the fixed forms; and (7) the humanistic vs. the materialistic. Sanders concludes her paper by asserting that "the critical question is not of African-American perspectives as much as it is of African-American participation and inclusion."

THE 1990 CONFERENCE ON
AFRICAN-AMERICAN PERSPECTIVES

The cumulative contributions from the 1987 Think Tank and the 1989 Conference led the steering committee to propose and to convene a conference in 1990 to explore more completely a set of philosophical issues regarded as essential for establishing the existence of African-American perspectives on biomedical ethics. The 1990 conference was cosponsored by Georgetown University, Howard University, Harvard University, and Glassboro State College with support from the Kaiser Family Foundation.

The essential issues or questions in the 1990 conference were the following: (1) Are there African-American perspectives on biomedical ethics, *an* African-American perspective, or *the* African-American Perspective: Cultural Relativism and Normative Issues: What are They? (2) What are the moral foundations of African and African-American cultures? (3) What is the African-American concept of personhood? and (4) What is the nature of wellness from African-American perspectives, and what are the roles of healers and patients in African and African-American cultures?

CULTURAL RELATIVISM

The major presentation for the first question was given by Jorge Garcia. Much of his discourse focuses on three aspects of Dr. Banner's 1989 thesis: (1) Does the realm of moral inquiry involve an extramental and extrapersonal order to things? (2) Does the concept of perspective have appropriate application within the realm of moral inquiry? and (3) Do human beings constitute a single moral and rational community?

Garcia's findings provide several assertions that will help clarify and direct the future work of this project. We can expect, for example, that there will be no single African-American perspective on issues such as biomedical ethics. He writes:

> While there is no acultural access to transcend the order of moral truth, there are facts about human beings, their nature and needs, origins and destiny that through cultural criticism, testing and sifting may provide us with a perspective on our moral life that is more comprehensive.

Garcia cites Dr. Sanders's theological claim that all theologies have a contextual point of departure rooted in the particularities of human experience. He also presents a listing and description of features that he thinks would make some perspectives on biomedical and applied ethics more meaningfully African-American. He points out that these are rooted in the elements of *source* (experience and standpoint); *content*, or how things might be regarded from an African-American viewpoint (anti-majoritarian, distrust, not bound to scientism), and *judgments*, which might ultimately influence practical and applied health care delivery issues.

Dr. Garcia concludes with a series of thoughts aimed at reforming, revising, and ultimately improving this project. He reminds us in agreeing with Sanders that our focus is on defining and articulating a human perspective that gives witness to universal truth.

To Garcia's treatment of the major issues in question number one, Tom Beauchamp and William Banner provide provocative, yet differing responses. Beauchamp begins his response with a discussion of relativism and continues with a catalog of what Garcia does and does not state in arriving at his position. Beauchamp concludes with an exploration of what he considers to be the uniqueness of African-American perspectives.

Banner's response to Garcia continues the discourse that he had initiated in 1989 when he posited his opposition to an ethnic perspective on biomedical ethics. In succinct and well-reasoned style, he does not waiver from his original position.

MORAL FOUNDATIONS

One of the consensus positions that emerged from the 1987 Think Tank was that African-Americans have emerged from historical and contemporary experiences that differ from those of other social groups within the United States. While Think Tank participants believed that the ethical principles of health care (e.g., autonomy, justice, beneficence) are the same for all, they believe that African-Americans invoke these principles differently, based on the unique historical experiences that have shaped their moral philosophy. Thus, the second question of the 1990 conference represents the exploration of assertions regarding cultural contributions to the development of moral philosophy. In order to approach this question, the steering committee wanted to examine the moral foundations of both African and African-American cultures.

Kwasi Wiredu, a philosopher and a native of Ghana, presents his reflections on the Akan people of his country. Beginning with an Akan philosophy of the human person, Wiredu proceeds to differentiate between notions of morals and religion. Having presented a conceptual understanding of morals and religion, he then considers the intellectual and personal aspects of human beings, i.e., their derivation and meaning. With a facile interweaving of these concepts, Wiredu lays before the reader the moral foundations of the Akan world view.

A number of Akanian maxims sprinkled throughout his paper provide an enriched purview of the moral foundation of the Akan culture, which are in turn translated by Wiredu into their practical application on the culture. The importance of the communalistic outlook as a ramification of Akan moral philosophy sheds light on that culture's approach to helping, dependency, kinship, aging, sex, and marriage.

As respondents to question number two, Robert Veatch and Marian Secundy provide the reader with several interesting notions. Veatch begins with an exploration of the moral foundations of African culture and proceeds to a discussion of normative ethics as applied to the conference question. He concludes with a discussion of the implications of an African-American biomedical ethics from a practical standpoint. Several of his concepts provide points of departure for further work in this area.

In her response to Wiredu's presentation, Secundy focuses on religious traditions as they apply to question number two. She provides several interesting connections between Africans and African-Americans in the United States.

CONCEPTS OF PERSONHOOD

The third question of the 1990 conference (the issue of personhood) actually emerged from the 1987 Think Tank. Three subsidiary issues

or questions had been raised: (1) How are African-Americans regarded as individuals? (2) How are they regarded in relation to other
groups or members of society? and (3) How is their status as persons
weighed when they are in competition for scarce resources? Kwasi
Wiredu and Laurence Thomas address this third question from African and African-American perspectives, respectively.

Wiredu takes a normative bent to the concept of person, again
employing examples and references to the Akan of Ghana. He describes the development of the person from conception to death and
beyond, using proverbs, as he had in the previous paper, to explain
Akan notions of personal freedom and responsibility. Finally, the critical constituents of the human being, i.e., the soul, the mind, and the
blood principle, are presented and described as important determinants of personhood and health among the Akan.

The second article that addresses the questions regarding personhood is one by Laurence Thomas entitled, "The Morally Beautiful."
To examine this question, Thomas looks at similarities or affinities between the African-American experience and the female experience in
arriving at the moral identity of self.

Thomas also concerns himself with responsibility, parental influence, the relationship between psychological and moral development, and choice. He uses his exploration of these concepts to arrive
at the position that in flourishing morally, a human being is at the
same time both vulnerable and in need of affirmation.

It is here that Thomas concludes his position vis-à-vis African-
Americans. He makes the case that despite being discounted morally
and intellectually, African-Americans have been affirmed as persons
largely through their nonverbal skills.

J. Bryan Hehir is the sole respondent to the Thomas and Wiredu
papers concerning question number three. Hehir begins his response
by sketching the development of similar concepts in Catholic Social
Ethics. Included in his discussion is the notion of rights and duties as
applied to conference question number three. Hehir concludes his
response with a discussion of three points of comparison between
themes found in the Wiredu and Thomas papers and Catholic notions
of rights and duties.

HEALTH CARE ISSUES

The fourth question of the 1990 conference: What is the nature of
health or wellness from an African-American perspective? and What
are the roles of healers and patients in African and African-American

cultures? was addressed in a two-part allegory by Leonard Harris. The reader is cautioned not to be overly entertained by the Harris paper as his philosophical positions are deeply rooted.

Harris delves into the concept of autonomy in the first part of his paper. He presents two views of autonomy: (a) independence and authenticity; and (b) independence with attendant constraint and respect. To deliver his first point he presents the allegory of Dr. Dick and his patient, George Washington Carver. The good doctor specialized in castration and abortion.

Throughout much of the first scenario, a debate is waged as to whether or not Dr. Dick should castrate his patient. The various ethical calculations engaged in by Dr. Dick and Carver's master provide a glimpse of the ridiculous and horrible realities experienced by many African-Americans in the health care system of the United States.

In his second allegory, Harris (and the reader) encounter Dr. Death, from whom Harris wants to procure services. As the allegory unfolds, Harris is unable to see Dr. Death or his assistant, Dr. Misery. Likewise, Dr. Goodbody, known for another type of service, is unavailable. Through discussions of the three physicians' services and characteristics, Harris begins his exploration of the fourth conference question.

Harris also discusses the concepts of autonomy and justice in the context of the social realities within which African-Americans encounter the health care system. For Harris, the background assumptions and intervening considerations that he discusses are key to his conception of ethical reasoning and, according to him, dominate the system.

Harris concludes his exploration of the fourth question by suggesting that African-Americans should continue to struggle with conceptions of health, ethos, and methodological applications. He ends his discourse with a strong statement on the importance of an African-American perspective on biomedical ethics.

Both Edmund Pellegrino and Lynn Peterson provide responses to Harris's paper. Pellegrino's response begins with a discourse on the need for a metacultural critique on bioethics and the implications emanating therefrom. His paper provides a formulation suggesting how such a critique should be constructed.

Peterson's response focuses on three issues raised in Harris's paper, namely, the conflicting roles and responsibilities of health care providers, when and how African-American perspectives should make a difference, and what can be learned if we teach the first two items.

OTHER MAJOR PAPERS

In addition to Dr. Banner's paper, two others from the 1989 Conference on African-American Perspectives on Biomedical Ethics are included in this volume. They are the papers of Cheryl Sanders and
James E. Bowman. The highlights of the Sanders paper have already
been discussed.

The Bowman manuscript begins with a philosophical exploration
of the "end of history" and its implications for the health of African-
Americans. He then discusses the effect of several diseases and conditions that influence the lives of African-Americans and the
technology used or misused in their treatment: Sickle Cell disease,
out of wedlock births, genetic disorders, and AIDS. He concludes
with a prognosis of how African-Americans may ultimately deal with
these and other conditions and the health care system.

Last but by no means least, this publication also includes the
keynote address delivered to the 1990 Conference by one of the few
remaining *homo universalis*, Herman Branson. In this address, Dr.
Branson eloquently reminds us of the hypothesis affirming the possibility that all civilization began in Africa. Branson also places great
importance on the value of trained intelligence and on a universal
ethic as keys to the conditions (health care systems included) that
bind African-Americans and all peoples in universal bondage.

It is in the spirit of Branson's universal ethic, that the reader is invited to partake of this text.

HARLEY FLACK

NOTES

1. See Edmund Pellegrino's response to Leonard Harris, "Culture and
Ethics: Need for a Metacultural Critique," in this volume.
2. See Emmet V. Mittlebeeler's Eurocentric analyses of colonialism's
"benefits" to traditional African society in *European Colonialism in Africa*
(Washington, D.C.: Georgetown University Press, 1961).
3. See Bill Moyers, *World of Ideas* (New York: Doubleday, 1989), p. 333.
4. Harley Flack, *Exploring Hospice: Caring and Critical Decision-Making*
(Unpublished manuscript, 1983).
5. *Think Tank on Black Perspectives in Biomedical Ethics* (Unpublished
proceedings from Georgetown University Kennedy Institute of Ethics,
February 11-13, 1987).
6. Cf. Aristotle, *On the Parts of Animals*, I.1.639a 20ff-639b.

Africa, African-Americans, and the Origin of a Universal Ethic

As a physics teacher, there have been innumerable times over the years when I have walked into a room confidently aware that I knew more about the topic than anybody in there. This a new experience tonight because I walk in here knowing that you know more about biomedical ethics, each and every one of you, than I do. I am essentially an amateur tonight, but not entirely. I have sat on the board of directors of the National Medical Fellowships for over thirty years, and on that board we have been concerned about black perspectives. . . . (You know, of course, that when I was growing up, we worked like the dickens to get people to call us negroes; then we moved on—color was acceptable, and we liked being called blacks, though I didn't quite get used to it myself. And now, you want me to use African-American. We'll have to be a little careful here. If I happen to use any one of those other terms, I am not being disrespectful, I am just exhibiting one of those wonderful conditions you cannot award, namely, that French condition called *agé* or A-G-E, which means that I find myself reverting sometimes to my former ways of doing things.)

Though I have been asked to give the keynote, my approach to the question of an African-American perspective on ethics may be too narrow. As I look back at all the philosophers I have read, I interpret them as saying that what we really seek is some great principle that African-Americans can grasp to aid them in mitigating some of the tragic conditions in this society. Now that may not be your concept of an African-American ethic, and it may not be mine when I get through, but it looks as though it may be a reasonable place to begin. We must of course guard against and be careful not to romanticize the subject—not to look on African-Americans as unique and different

1

human beings. We are not. Each and every one of us, like all people everywhere has between thirty billion and a hundred billion neurons in the brain. I'd like to think that we have a few more than most people, but that's not allowed. Those are the tools with which we have to operate. But remember that most of those neurons are given to thinking about very pedestrian things, because one's body is a fantastically complex mechanism. Some energy has got to say, "Okay, cell, now you divide; okay, cell, now you die." And you don't consciously take time for that, because you're trying to figure out the simple things like what are we going to have for dinner. So the body for the most part does those things on autopilot. We are blessed.

Human beings are the only creatures, seemingly, in the universe—at least we have no evidence of any others—who are conscious of themselves and self-projecting. Now in recent years we have gained some fantastic insights, primarily due to scientists in the last half-century who have provided us with instruments for looking at the universe. I remember a day in February, 1987. A light flashed in the heavens that wasn't there the day before, a supernova. Everybody was excited who heard about this new thing only to learn that the supernova did not occur on that February night, but 160,000 years before its light reached us. Don't you admire the creature, the human being, who can learn those things? And don't you disdain the same creature, the same human being, who can't keep little babies from dying in our cities, in Philadelphia, New York and Washington, D.C.? Somehow we have got to find solutions, and that is something you and I and everyone will have to do together.

Now in all the history of human beings, Africa is surely a fascinating country. Sir Thomas Brown (ca. 1600) said, "We carry within us the wonder we seek without us. There is all Africa and her prodigies in us." That is a great statement. And recent scientific developments—some in the last three years—have tapped this wonder.

First, consider the notion that human beings, and all mammals really, have male and female origins. The male contributes a spermlike bit that doesn't have enough sense to go right in. It just gets there and puts its head in. The female then contributes an egg, a big, nutritious medium. The sperm goes in, primarily with genetic materials; the egg from the female carries the life mechanisms and the energy sources we call the mitochondria. Each and every one of us gets his or her mitochondria from the mother.

A beautiful thing, no? That we can trace life's energy right on back to "mama, mama, mama." Once it is said that the mother contributes more than the father in procreation, doesn't it follow, therefore, that in every divorce proceeding she should have precedence? We may be hearing this argument soon.

The mitochondria is very important, but it is also a relatively simple molecule. And hanging on to it, so to speak, are Alpha helixes of amino acids, and those amino acids will mutate. To mutate is a high-faluting word for "change," and scientists estimate that a two to four percent mutation in amino acids happens every million years. A research team in California made an alarmingly fascinating discovery. They looked at the mitochondria from 147 people from all over the world, using this mutation rate. They looked and saw that certain of these amino acids had indeed mutated. This is a well-known fact. For example, sickle-cell anemia is caused by the joining of a hemoglobin molecule in position six to a glutamic acid, which is in that position normally. They become a valine, and that minute change creates havoc. How many amino acid diseases stem from such small mutations? Well, sickle-cell anemia is one such disease that I thought could be immediately resolved, but it hasn't been. And that is where we stand.

As scientists looked at the mitochondria in all these peoples, they made charts. They looked, and they plotted, and the whole thing seemed to point right back to one late afternoon in Africa's great rift valley, a beautiful place. Everyone should go to Africa. Everybody ought to see the rift valley, because as you stand on its edge and look down, you can almost visualize your great, great, great grandmother. She must have been a powerful woman, this mother of us all. She could not have been a sniveling female. This was a real woman. Again, you look down and your information converges to a time roughly 200,000 years ago and the evidence is very convincing that Eve was the woman in the great rift valley who gave her mitochondria to everybody, to all human beings on this earth.

Now needless to say, there are people who don't want to believe this simple thing, and many who are never going to believe it; but the idea is in the forefront. Hardbone anthropologists don't like it; they think it can't be right. But the evidence is extremely convincing that Africa is, in a certain sense, the mother of us all.

The wonderful things that come out of Africa! Oh, you know the statement. I remember when I studied Latin, I could only translate short sentences—*Ex Africa . . . Sempre alii quid Novi*—"what are all the good new things always coming out of Africa?" Pliny said that before the year 100. And this notion, that all humankind, not just African-Americans but all of us, are members of the same family is entirely consistent with the major premises of African humanism.

The main tenet of African humanism is that all people are children of the same God. Now just change the phrase slightly to say that all people are children of the same mother, that wonderful African woman of 200,000 years ago! But knowing this doesn't make everything wonderful right now. It does no good to tell everybody that we are children of the same mother: no one is going to respond, "My brother, come right here, and we will welcome you." We know that that is not true. For there is another sort of background that we also share that we can call a database of neglect.

I should mention here two or three issues that I think we must include in our observations. A recent issue of *American Health*—a very good article for our purposes—claims that roughly, in 1987, 255,000 African-Americans died, and of those 255,000 who died, 75,000 would not have died except for neglect. If all the factors making for health and protection had been applied to African-Americans, 75,000 of them would not have died in 1987, according to my calculations. Then I looked at the death rate for everyone. An article in the *Journal of the American Medical Association* suggests that one-third of the 75,000 deaths can be attributed to high blood pressure, high cholesterol, obesity, diabetes, smoking, and drinking; and another third, to low income. Finally—and I like this category— the author says that one third of these 75,000 deaths are from the stress of racism. I never heard anybody quantify such stress before. Yet I know it exists. If a medical man of some reputation says these things, then you must see what we are up against.

Consider further the middle category of these causes of premature death. A low-income person will die of neglect. That news is available in the *New York Times*; if any African-American goes to a hospital in New York City, he or she does not get the highest level of attention or medicine. Attention, yes, but too little, of too little quality. And certainly, many poor women, in New York and elsewhere, leave the hospitals having received inadequate care, and many more die of breast cancer. These deaths, too, are caused by low income.

Not that the African-American should only be concerned about the immediate. Remember that we are in the midst of one of the most desperate periods in the history of humankind. What do I mean by that? As you know our population is aging. At the beginning of this century life expectancy was 47; now it's about to level off at nearly 80. But 80-year-olds are not as socially effective as 30-year-olds and the job of taking care of this aging population will give us many, many difficulties.

A second point is the tremendous increase in our population. I remember my great grandmother. She was born in 1850, and now here I am at 70, some 140 years later. My great grandmother spoiled me, and I thank her very, very, much; I am beholden to her for much. But the important thing is this: in 1850, there were only a billion people on the earth. And now, before the death of her great grandson, there are five billion people—a fivefold increase in 140 years. Suppose that goes on; in 130 or 140 years from now, in the year 2130, then how many people will we have? 25 billion. It can't be. It can't be. We've got to think carefully about controlling such increases.

We need to assess the disturbances. For example, if we look at the earth in terms of renewable resources, we discover that the earth is not a bottomless cavern of goodies. As a matter of fact, look at only one of the commodities that we must have, namely, water. Experts tell us that we have only enough water for 9 billion people. Before our lifespan is finished, we may be without sufficient water. Now we can solve that problem with fusion energy—not fission energy, but fusion energy. Fission energy rightfully scares the life out of human beings. It should.

Remember Chernobyl and the trouble it caused? My wife and I were in Russia recently, and we discovered that the defective reactor has been sealed. But three or four other reactors in that Chernobyl complex are going lickety-split. They are going lickety-split because human beings have concluded, "Okay, if we cut them off, we will have no energy, no food, and we will die. If we keep them, they may explode and kill us, but we will have lived a little longer anyway." Fission energy is efficient energy.

But there is another source of energy. And it's tragic that Western and Russian physicists are not applying themselves to it. Fusion energy is what the sun does. The sun has the ability, the fantastic ability, to take four nuclei of hydrogen, fuse them into one nucleus of helium, and mass the effect to turn them into energy. That's how the sun shines. If the sun hadn't fused hydrogen and helium; if the sun were pure anthracite, burning in an atmosphere of pure oxygen, it would only burn at its present rate for about seven thousand years.

It required an odd, odd mechanism to make the sun shine, and this is it. The oceans are a great source of hydrogen. If we could use them to produce fusion energy, we would have clean energy way into the future. Survival is a race to find clean energy, and to make it available for all the peoples on this earth. But it won't happen. I think that we are not concerned enough. We do not yet know that "Chernobyls" are too dangerous for human beings.

Here, then, are the kinds of programs we must have. But when we turn to medicine we are struck dumb because medicine is really such a strange field—though perhaps I shouldn't say anything like that, standing so close to my distinguished former student, the Dean of Howard Medical School. Truthfully, however, does it not take a great genius to conquer medicine? One of the reasons simple people like me are apt to ignore a great deal of medicine is that it does not ensure longevity. One can go places where nothing special is being done in the way of health, and find there a woman or man who lives to be 105 or 127 years old, while someone else, in Washington, D.C., dies at 38. Each of us has Walter Mitty spells. I remember how, once when I wanted something I couldn't have, I envied Mr. Nelson Rockefeller, who had all the money in the world. Suddenly he is dead, and I am still here. There is something wrong.

Thus, the idea that medicine does not ensure longevity. But medicine does relieve pain, and will relieve pain, if only it is properly used. We have seen the figures—47 years' life expectancy in 1900; 80 years in 1991—though some people are always critical on this issue. In 1976 Ivan Illych wrote a very interesting book called *The Limits of Medicine*, and I have just seen a new one (1990) by Daniel Callahan, called *What Kind of Life: The Limits of Medical Progress*. These critical assessments of medicine are worth knowing; they do not mean, however, that poor people need no medicine. We can never say that because there are painful "conditions," infections, in life that must be treated, whether or not the treatment increases life expectancy. Some even contend that modern medicine came into existence in 1954 or 1956, when Sulfonamides were introduced.

What, then, can we think about an African-American perspective? First, we must remember that African-Americans may not be put down as a single unity, the views of certain philosophers notwithstanding. I looked into Hegel on this point, specifically into his discussion about the *volksgeist*. According to him, the *volksgeist* develops only if a people have the same history. Well, you won't find such uniformity among African-Americans.

Some years ago, when I was just starting my career, a man by the name of Melville Herskowitz, who was a very able sociologist at Northwestern University, and a student of blacks, that is, African-Americans, found that out of 3,300 African-American students, there were only 300 or 400 who did not carry mixed genes, who did not also have Native American and white genes and perhaps others. African-Americans have evolved in America as a separate group with a genetic tie to all people. But, again, society does not permit us to decide which of our genetic ties we shall announce ourselves as beholden to.

Malcolm X tells a story about the young African-American he met at Harvard who had just taken his Ph.D. He was feeling rather good—as was his right—and said to Malcolm X, "You know, Malcolm, I wonder what they call me?" And Malcolm said, "Nigger." In other words, no matter where we are, no matter what our genetic combination may be, we are still subject to oppression. Such realizations should make us work more closely to alleviate not only our own condition but also to aid Africa, which may be, perhaps, the major source of our genes.

What, then, can we say of our African heritage? It, too, is not experienced as a univocal force. I have been on the council of the National University of Lesotho for the last six years. I go to Johannesburg and to Lesotho each March, and there I learned that South Africa publishes books for Africans in at least eight different languages: Norosto, Sorsoto, Desuana, the Dinnguy languages, Zulu, Chosa, Swazi, and others. Such richness may be looked at in two ways: it is wonderful to respect the cultures of those young people, but so many translations may also continue a certain divisiveness.

Divisiveness is so much easier than unity, but what can be done? I don't think there is any easy solution. Africans do not all speak the same language. People around the Cape in South Africa, the estimated 2.5 million "coloreds" as they are called, learn Afrikaans and some English in school. Therefore, they are unable to talk to the Africans. You never find anyone in Capetown who can speak Zulu or any tribal languages and that makes for some of the difficulty. Even those who are in a group of closely related languages, for example, the Inguny languages of Zulu and Chosa, are divided. Zulu means man, and if you are not a Zulu, with your name spelled and pronounced like a Zulu name, then you are not a man; and you will have grave difficulties speaking with a Zulu. This is a problem we must work to alleviate. It is not impossible: when we return to America and reflect on this problem, we find there are alternatives. The end to divisiveness may have to begin with us and with nonlinguistic questions.

One way to begin may be with those figures I gave you about needless death among African-Americans. Those figures can, and most assuredly should be improved. I think, moreover, that the improvement can be made despite the expensive technology of modern medicine. Not everybody needs the most expensive technology. Of course, we have the attitude that if we are in the hospital, and the hospital is up-to-date, then we want the very latest—the CAT scan, for example. In Great Britain, only six women out of 1,000 have hysterectomies; here in North America, the number is 50 or 60 out of 1,000. Why? Well, perhaps our doctors like to perform this surgery, regardless of whether it is the most effective intervention.

And now, I will review and conclude with a story, for we cannot review and conclude without recognizing that although diversity exists everywhere in Africa, it is extremely traumatic. Recently there was a wonderful—not wonderfully good but wonderfully bad—health care situation in Kenya. Kenya is a very attractive country.

Nairobi, Kenya, for example, has probably the best climate in the world. The Kukuyu and the Luo are two of Kenya's largest tribes. When I first went to the University of Nairobi, everybody I met was a Kukuyu. When I got to the Vice Chancellor, I said, "Are you a Kukuyu?" He said, "Oh yes, I am a Kukuyu. But remember a lot of Kukuyu's are in jail, too." He told me that.

Now recently a Kukuyu lady married a Luo man who was a distinguished lawyer with money and family. But the Kukuyu and the Luo differ radically in the way they look at death and in the way they interpret family responsibilities. The Luo man said, "I want to be buried in Nairobi on my farm." His family hit the ceiling. "You can't do that," they told him, "you must be buried with your people."

The Kukuyu are very bright and speak very fast. They are involved in every argument. The Kukuyu wife alienated many people by the things she said. Eventually the court decided that the man's body should go back to his family. But the case revealed that even in a small country like this, there are very disparate attitudes toward living and dying—toward respect paid to the dead—and even the Kukuyu seem to ignore the dead sometimes.

Nevertheless, Africa has always enjoyed high esteem in peoples' opinions. One description that was new to me was written by Keats in the 1800s. He said, "Son of the old moon mountain—Africa." We African-Americans may want to call ourselves "sons of the old moon mountain." If so, the rest of America can say, "I'm a friend of the son of the old moon mountain."

Shakespeare also loved Africa. Did you know that? I didn't know that. In Henry IV, Part II, he wrote, "I speak of Africa and golden joys." He was describing love for Africa and the opinion that Africans are good people who are worthy of respect, admiration and attention.

So, after going at the topic in this fashion, where do I end up? Remember, a physics teacher has always to come down to a specific problem. I tried to find a philosopher whose ideas would encapsulate all the concerns we have for Africa, and all the things that we must do for African-Americans. But in the end, perhaps only one thing is certain: the conditions of modern life. The rule is absolute: the race that does not value trained intelligence is doomed. I would like to tell you that I made that up, but it was Alfred North Whitehead who said it some years ago. Still, it is very significant for the African-American, because our problems are not going to be solved by pure devotion; they will be solved only if we bring to bear on them the highest quality of trained intelligence. If we do that, then when the negative occasions arise, we can say, "Hey, wait a minute. Don't go off shooting people. Don't support these horrible ethnic and religious clashes that are now taking place." Ask yourself instead how these problems can be resolved. It is not going to be easy.

It is a terrible thing when somebody is gunned down for having different ideas and different approaches to things. Don't believe, for example, that African-Americans are stigmatized because of their color. The Japanese have a group whom they call the Etas, a really oppressed group in Japan; but if you look at them, you cannot tell an Eta from any other Japanese. Their physiognomy is normal, but they were stigmatized years ago because they did the dirty jobs: they cleaned the latrines; they slaughtered the animals; they cured the leper. The stigma continues even though the law since 1877 has forbidden it.

The Japanese keep very, very detailed and deep family records. If a charming young lady meets a charming young man and decides to get married, immediately the family background is investigated. If the man or woman is an Eta, the other family will oppose the marriage. Suicides are committed—a very harsh judgment indeed. The Japanese claim to be getting away from such nonsense, but I am told that it still persists. We are not in Japan; possibly we cannot solve this problem for them.

We can, however, do one useful thing, if nothing else, when our circumstances are similarly belittled, and our history and worth as human beings are held up to ridicule. We can remember who is the one dishonored by prejudice. There is an old Bantu saying: "The African is like an Indian rubber ball; the harder you dash him to the ground, the higher he jumps." That sounds nice, doesn't it? It's not true, of course. But you can say it. It means that the African is hearty, though he or she should not be punished and cannot be overcome.

I urge you to think, throughout this meeting and forever, that the major ethic (singular) that African-Americans can seize on and carry forward is an intense respect for, and dedication to, trained intelligence. If we do that, we are apt to move through this society doing and achieving those things that are needed: raising more questions with more data more often about why certain things are done. The moral question is not that 75,000 African-Americans die in any given year but that 75,000 African-Americans die who should not have died! That's what we have to do something about.

I will give you an example. In 1970, a group of African-American college presidents called on Mr. Nixon, and I prepared what I thought was a very good statement lambasting the federal government for not doing something more for the historically black colleges. After I had read it, Mr. Nixon turned to Mr. Allen who was commissioner of education and said, "Jim, is this true?" He said, "I'm afraid it is, Mr. President." And Mr. Nixon said, "Well that's a damn shame; I'm going to do something about it." And he did. He gave $120 million the following year to Title III—an immense help to the black colleges. What is important here is that if we had merely been outside the White House picketing the administration (though mind you, somebody had to be out there picketing), little would have been accomplished. Instead, we went to the table with data, and some progress was made. When we told Nixon the facts, he couldn't say, "Oh, don't worry, you get all you deserve."

The same tactic, however, did not work so well before the legislature in Pennsylvania. There I pointed out that the median income of African-American families is roughly 60 percent of the median income of white families, therefore, of the four state-related universities (Lincoln, Penn State, Temple, and Pittsburgh), Lincoln's costs should be no more than 60 percent of the costs at those other institutions. Richard Thornburg, a good friend and a gentleman, knew our cause was a good one, but the state didn't give us the money. The point is not that we will always win, but that we must have a valid argument.

Let this be the thing we do in the name of an African-American ethic: Dedication to trained intelligence—learning, knowing, moving, doing, presenting. For then the future will be significantly brighter, and honor will be done to the fact that most of our genes come from Africa. I found a magnificent Yoruba statement to guide us. It reads: "Only the things for which you have struggled will last."

HERMAN BRANSON, PH.D.

Jorge L. A. Garcia

African-American Perspectives, Cultural Relativism, and Normative Issues: Some Conceptual Questions

My project here is to deal with the conceptual questions embedded in this discussion of African-American perspectives on biomedical ethics. Specifically, I want to explore and to sketch the rudiments of some answers to these questions: (1) What is it for a position on an ethical issue to reflect (involve) an ethnic perspective? (2) How is an ethnic perspective on such issues possible? (3) What would be the good of such a perspective? and (4) What dangers or limitations might attend its acknowledgement and utilization?

William Banner has made this task at once easier and more difficult. Easier, because he has helped us see more clearly the questions that need to be answered; more difficult, because the issues he raises are so complex. Banner argues against the possibility of any "ethnic perspective in medical science and in ethics," insisting that "there is only one medical community, which address itself to the alleviation of physical and mental discomfort and disease, and one ethical or moral community, which addresses itself to the responsibilities of good judgment, justice, and compassion." In ethics, he maintains, we "encounter . . . an extramental, extrapersonal order of things to which the term 'perspective' is inapplicable or inappropriate," and thus "the conduct of the science of ethics is incompatible with anything called an 'ethnic perspective.'" He qualifies this sweeping judgment only to the extent of adding that "if we are to use the term 'perspective' at all, we must . . . speak of the rational and humane perspective."[1]

It appears, then, that three claims constitute the heart of Banner's challenge to those who think it makes sense to talk about ethnic perspectives—African-American or otherwise—on any normative field. These three claims are as follows: (B1) The realm of moral

11

inquiry involves an extramental and extrapersonal order of things. (B2) The concept of perspective has no appropriate application within such a realm. (B3) Human beings constitute a single moral and rational community, membership in which affords them all a single rational and humane perspective on moral issues.

I wish to sketch three lines of response to the challenge that Banner's theses pose, arguing against the first, endorsing the second, and taking no firm stance on the last.

CULTURAL RELATIVISM, THE FIRST RESPONSE

Cultural relativists deny all three theses, but it will serve our purposes to concentrate on their denial of the first thesis (B1). Banner doesn't specify what he means to exclude by calling an order "extramental" and "extrapersonal," so I will take the liberty of stipulating that we have entered an extramental order when the truth (or objective warrant) of judgments in that order is not wholly derivative from the preferences and impressions, that some individuals or groups happen to have.[2] Cultural relativists deny that the moral realm is extramental in this sense, because they see that realm as a personal order in which groups of people organize their lives together by expressing, acting from, and inculcating such shared mental responses such disapproval, shame, or guilt. From this vision of the moral realm, it follows that, insofar as humans comprise different groups, there is not one moral community but many; and that "perspective," understood as a standpoint from within some group, is a pervasive and inescapable feature of moral judgment.

We can understand cultural relativism, in the forms with which we are concerned, as essentially involving three theses: (1) a *relativity* thesis, holding that some moral judgments are somehow relative to the codes or lifestyles of cultural groups; (2) a *diversity* thesis, holding that these codes or lifestyles are not entirely identical in what they commend, enjoin, and so on; and (3) a *nonrankability* thesis, restricting the extent to which different codes, or opposed provisions drawn from different codes, can be ordered as better or worse.[3] Each of these elements affords a dimension, which I shall label judgmental scope, depth, and strength, respectively, in respect to which any two relativist moral views can vary.

Regarding the first thesis, consider the view of a person who endorses some form of cultural relativism but thinks it doesn't apply to judgments about justice.[4] That makes her relativism less extensive in scope than that of someone who holds *all* moral judgments to be relativized. Regarding the second, consider the claim that some types of behavior—for example, killing a group-member's children just for fun—are disallowed in every culture. This kind of claim is attractive to those who join to their relativism the functionalist belief that the purpose of a moral code is to harmonize the pursuit of individual interests within the group.[5] Such a position displays a relativism that doesn't go as deep as that found in the view that there are no such (cross-culturally) universal moral norms.

Regarding the third, consider the position of someone who, while she thinks that morality is just a matter of a group's code and that codes differ in content from group to group, nonetheless maintains that there are some nonmoral standards that can legitimately serve as a nonrelativized basis for saying that the code of, say, Group Number One is better than is that of Group Number Two. Any relativist who also holds the functionalist belief mentioned above would seem to be thereby *committed* to the existence of such nonrelativized bases for evaluating codes, since some group's code may fulfill these functions, for example, insuring the survival of its group's culture, less effectively than some other group's code. Such a relativism is not so strong as that of someone who insists that no nonrelativized standards exist by which different codes can properly be evaluated.

Alain Locke's relativism and value pluralism

This last view, that the moral codes of diverse societies cannot be ranked as better and worse, calls to mind the writings of Alain Locke, who has been called "the most-noted Afro-American philosopher to date," and who describes himself as "philosophical mid-wife to a generation of younger Negro poets, writers, [and] artists."[6] Locke condemned the "value bigotry" he thought accompanied "value absolutism." Against it, he advocated what he called a form of "value pluralism" and tied this to "social reciprocity," by which, according to one sympathetic commentator, Locke meant "that groups must share values; value-groups, cultural groups, and ethnic groups must give and receive from each other so that each may enrich the other. In this way, he hoped, the myths of value superiority and the attitudes that promote . . . racism could be dispelled. . . ."[7] In Locke's own words, "social reciprocity for value loyalties is but a new name for the old virtue of tolerance. . . . Relativism will have to slowly tame the wild force of our imperatives."[8]

In fact, Locke's moral thought is quite complex and I cannot claim to fathom the exact relativism he held or why he held it. He thinks that experience in each of the four fields of value he identifies, the religious, the moral, the logical, and the aesthetic, derives from its own characteristic mode of feeling in the individual—feelings of exaltation, tension, agreement, and repose, respectively. In this way, "values are rooted in attitudes, not in reality, and pertain to ourselves, not to the world." Recognition of this subjective origin of value might prove an "effective antidote to value absolutism" and enable us to develop a type of "value loyalty" independent of "value bigotry."[9] He insists, however, that "this type of value pluralism does not invite the chaos of value anarchy, "because we can still be loyal to our values, and even to the imperatives associated with them, by accepting some norms as "functional and native to the process of experience," and by accepting the imperatives as "categorical," as he puts it, "without calling down fire from heaven. Norms of this status," he explains, "would be functional constants and practical sustaining imperatives of their correlated modes of experience."[10]

There is much that is valuable in Locke's value theory, particularly in his suggestive remark that each of the modes of emotional response that grounds an experience of value admits both an introverted and extroverted type, by means of which he hoped to clarify the nature of the strife between the mystic and the reformer in religion, between the mathematically-inclined and the experimentally-inclined in the sciences, and even between the critic and the creator in the arts.[11] Locke's axiological thought may well be a chest of unexplored treasures.

Locke's espousal of a relativistic type of value pluralism, however, is a different matter. As we saw, his value theory begins in the subject's mind, but then is somehow broadened so as to admit functional values and even categorical imperatives. The claims that a plurality of values exists and that we need to guard against excessive loyalty to some values over others are introduced as claims about different fields of value—religious, moral, logical, and aesthetic—not as claims about different systems of value judgments *within* the same field.

> Even after lip service to the parity of Beauty, Truth, and Good, we conspire for the priority of one pet favorite, which usually reflects merely our dominant value interest and our temperamental value bias. The growth of modern relativism has at least cooled these erstwhile burning issues. . . .[12]

Cultural pluralism, relativism, and tolerance of values enter Locke's picture in a more problematical way. Having affirmed, without much argument, the parity of the four fields of value and the need to guard against the tendency of any one of the four corresponding modes of value feeling to monopolize our experience of value to the exclusion of the other modes, he finds in this parity and this need for toleration "warrant for our taking as the center of value loyalty neither the worship of definitions nor the competitive monopolizing of value claims, but the goal of maximizing the value-mode itself as an attitude and activity."[13] If I understand him, Locke then interprets this maximization so as to counsel the multiplication of conflicting value-systems, including, presumably, a variety of contesting aesthetic movements, different religious denominations, opposed moral beliefs and practices, and perhaps even varying scientific methodologies and theories.

It is hard to discern Locke's line of reasoning here. Plainly, he meant his endorsement of maximization to contrast with "the competitive monopolizing of value claims" that he had previously criticized. In its original context, however, competitive monopolizing referred to the supposed inclination of values in one field, for example, religious ones, to be so demanding as to thwart our cultivation or appreciation of values in other fields.[14] That position implies nothing about whether a plurality of competing views about morality or holiness might be a good thing, as Locke seems to infer.

What of the other position that Locke rejects in the passage cited, that "the proper center of value loyalty" might lie in "the worship of definitions and formulae"? This rhetoric is powerful, but it is difficult to say the same for the reasoning. He seems to be referring here to an inordinate attachment to or worship of particular positions or systems of thought within a field of values, for example, the credo of a religious denomination or of a specific aesthetic movement (such as the Negritude movement).[15] But, again, contrary to what Locke says, there is no "warrant" for this dismissal of particular value attachments in the plurality and parity of fields of values he has earlier affirmed. Even if, for the sake of argument, we grant Locke his implausible premise that there is parity among the fields of value (that religious values, say, are neither higher nor lower than aesthetic ones), that in no way warrants his conclusion that the different specific and opposed positions *within* a field are likewise all on a par.

The strongest ground for such a latitudinarian conclusion that I can find in Locke's text is this claim: "As creatures of a mode of experience, they [the assorted fields of value] should not construe themselves in any concrete embodiment so as to contradict or stultify the mode of which they are a particularized expression."[16] Even this does not make a very strong case. At most, it shows that we should reject a particular system of, for example, moral values, if that system thwarts our ability to experience the very type of value feeling in which such values originate. Locke offers no reason to assume, however, that every particular system of moral values (to keep our focus on the moral) will thwart the type of value feelings from which it arises; and certainly it is unlikely that every particular system should thwart those feelings to the same extent. This claim, then, even if true, provides little grounds for the proposition Locke apparently wants to use in order to ground his principle of cross-cultural moral toleration: the proposition that all particular systems of moral value are on a par.

Assessing cultural relativism

Whatever the rationale behind Alain Locke's version of relativism, there are serious problems confronting any form of cultural relativism that is significantly extensive, deep or strong in its judgmental scope. There is no reason to call any set of judgments or practices in a society moral judgments or practices unless they are recognizable as such. And, of course, we can recognize them as moral only insofar as they pertinently resemble what we ordinarily call moral. But this pits some of the cultural relativists' claims against others, especially as their relativism becomes more extensive and deeper in judgmental scope. They need the judgments and practices in question to be similar enough to our own to be recognizable as moral, but they also need them to be different enough from our own to support the relativity thesis. Nor will it do for relativists to say that these judgments differ from ours in content but are similar in the rationale supporting them, for this will mean that relativism evaporates as we approach the deeper moral claims that serve as the epistemic or justificatory basis of our judgments or practices. At that point, the cultural relativists' best hope is to insist on some purely formal criteria for recognizing moral judgments and practices. But formalism, too, is problematic in the light of the philosophical criticism of the last few decades and, in any case, merely begs the question against those who hold that nothing should be counted as a moral judgment or practice unless it is similar in subject, content, and rationale to the only paradigms we have of the moral, that is, to the judgments we ordinarily make, the practices in which we ordinarily participate.[17]

There is an additional problem besetting the formalist's way out. The most common and appealing purely formal criteria of the moral are those that select a judgment or practice as moral only if it serves a certain social end, such as the survival of the group's unity or its members' lives. As we noted above, however, any strong nonrankability thesis is implausible in functionalist forms of relativism, since such forms have, built into whatever function they take as definitive of moral codes, a nonrelativized standard for evaluating such codes.[18] The formalist who rejects functionalism may instead try to identify a society's moral judgments as those that trigger such responses as guilt, shame, praise, blame, and ostracism. This procedure, however, is likely to prove circular. Moral judgments must be tied to moral guilt or moral blame. But there is no way to tell if this person's guilt or that one's blame is moral guilt or blame unless we can already recognize that the judgments on which it is based are moral judgments. Clearly, then, we cannot rely on our recognition of moral guilt to identify moral judgments.

Cultural relativists may want to restrict the judgmental scope of their relativism, retreating to a position like that of some recent philosophers who maintain that relativism applies to assessments of personal ideals and social "ways of life," but exempting judgments about justice from its scope.[19] There are reasons for pessimism about such a strategy's prospects. It seems likely, for example, that your right to my assistance in securing health care grows less stringent as the assistance becomes more onerous for me, interfering with my legitimate ideals and way of life. But this means that the correctness of a judgment about the legitimacy of a way of life (a relativized judgment, on the view in question) will depend on a judgment of justice (a nonrelativized judgment), and vice versa. Perhaps this can be worked out, but it seems to me that this sort of interdependence of judgments of justice with judgments about ways of life will make it very difficult to segregate the two kinds of moral judgment in the way that this limited-scope cultural relativism requires.

It may be objected to my argument that it is Eurocentric, taking the moral judgments and practices of some Western cultures to be normative in that no other culture's judgments or practices are to be counted as moral unless they sufficiently resemble the Western paradigm. There is, of course, some truth to this objection, but I don't see it as very damaging to my argument. First, the "Eurocentrism" is not essential but is merely a function of the fact that we are speaking a Western tongue and asking in it a question about what has to be true of a judgment or practice for us to apply to it the English term, "moral," which term picks out certain concepts that, even if they arose in Africa or Asia, have developed in a peculiar way in the West. In an exactly parallel way, a Polynesian asking whether modern Americans have a code of *tabu* must determine whether anything in this society closely enough matches the *tabu* that she is familiar with in Polynesian culture to warrant saying that modern American society also has such a code. Thus, while there is an essential element of the ethnocentric in the methodology, there is nothing essentially *Eurocentric* in it.

Second, as I have just pointed out, the ethnocentrism is merely methodological, and even here it lies mainly in the starting point. This may be disappointing to those who, like certain optimists with Cartesian leanings, think they can begin their scholarly inquiries from some neutral territory unmarked by the folkways of any particular cultural tradition. The point, however, is merely the familiar one that Alain Locke imbibed from his pragmatist teachers at Harvard: there are no presuppositionless starting points; we must begin from where we are. That means that when we look for the term and concept of "the moral," we must begin with the English term and the particular concept it expresses, given its historical development in Western tongues and thought.

It would, of course, be foolhardy to suppose that the arguments I've offered serve to refute all forms of cultural relativism, and I make no such claim.[20] I do think, however, that they indicate that any form of relativism that is strong, deep, and extensive in its judgmental scope, will suffer from such internal tensions as to render it an unappealing line of response to Banner's challenge. To these internal tensions plaguing all forms of relativism we may, by the way, add another that affects Alain Locke's effort to link relativism to a principle of cross-cultural tolerance. Unless he means his relativism to be much less extensive than his rhetoric suggests, Locke is in no position to claim for tolerance any other status than it has as simply another local value of certain cultural traditions.[21] It is not at all clear on what basis Locke could argue even that Westerners should put greater store in tolerance than they invest in other items from their stock of values, such as individualism (or, for that matter, monotheism). Aside from the question of how he could argue for that position, it is unclear how he could so much as endorse it without contradicting his own relativistic brand of value pluralism.

INTERPRETING PERSPECTIVES REALISTICALLY, A SECOND RESPONSE

A second line of response denies the middle thesis in Banner's challenge, that is, the thesis that if morality involves an extramental, extrapersonal order of things, then the concept of perspective is inapplicable to it (B2). A little reflection should reveal that this is a very odd thesis indeed. The realm of experience that the term "perspective" first calls to mind, the realm indicated in the very root and prefix of the word itself, is that of vision. A perspective, as one dictionary has it, is a "manner in which things appear to the eye in respect to their relative positions and distance."[22] The dictionary entry captures the essentials, I think, but it omits some alterations that a change in one's perspective, a shift of vantage points, will bring. Take a cylindrical cup, three inches deep. As you hold it up before your eyes, it looks larger than the sun. But if you set the same cup a few feet away on a tabletop, its rim will appear ovoid when you look at it. Further, we know that the parallel lines in its exterior decoration would, if you set the cup on its side, sighted along the lines, and extended them to the horizon, appear to meet. These are the commonplace phenomena of changed visual perspectives on physical objects.

When we bear these observations in mind, Banner's second thesis is quite puzzling. Plainly, if there is any order of things beyond the mind and person, then the visual perception of the attributes of figure and extension must involve it. Excepting philosophers in the grip of metaphysical idealism, no one will maintain that the truth of a judgment about a figure's length, width, height, or shape is wholly derived from the preferences or impressions of any individual or group. Yet this realm of phenomena is not only *compatible* with talk of perspectives, it is the very realm in which such talk originates and is used most literally.

What we encounter here is one of the oldest of philosophical topics—the difference between appearance and reality. The cup's rim *is* round but from a certain perspective *looks* elliptical. Changes in perspective affect appearances, not reality. Of course, the nature of the relationship between appearance and reality has long been a matter of philosophical controversy.

In the West, especially in the epoch of modernism, many metaphysicians have sought to understand how things really are, their objective attributes, as somehow constructed out of the way things appear. Primarily, they have wanted to construct the objective order out of the *inter*subjective, construing the way an object *is* as, roughly, the way it appears to people in a self-consistent way as they move through different times and places. Thus, we gather perceptual information about how an object O looks at time t to a subject $S1$ who is located at place $P1$ and similar information about how, at the same time, it appears to subject $S2$ who is located at place $P2$, and soon, we approach a conception of how the object appears from nowhere in particular. In this way of looking at the construction of our understanding of reality, we move from the content of subjective perception to the concept of the object and the objective realm. This is then taken somehow to constitute (or to be the basis for constructing) a concept of how the object *objectively is* (that is, how it is as an object *of experience*, and not simply of any one subject's isolated experience of it).[23]

The cognitive process whereby we come to articulate perceptual knowledge is thus a pervasively *human* one. It is fashioned, first, by the perceiver's biochemistry, but it is also true that the language in which she expresses her claims about the qualities she perceives in things will have arisen in some human society, and even the concepts internal to her knowing (for example, such notions as red or square) will have been shaped by her culture's history and needs. (Whether a certain surface should be called red or orange, for example, is a matter of linguistic conventions that may leave the answer indeterminate and which themselves arose in response to historical forces.) Nothing, however, in these features of human knowing shows that the world, the facts, she comes to know are merely hers, or merely ours. Even if our knowing is a deeply human matter, we have no reason to think that the world itself, or the facts of which it is "the totality," is merely a human construct.[24] It remains open to say that it is simply *the* world—open to everyone to understand as best she can, helped and hindered as she will be by various features of her culture and her chemistry.

Elements for a perspectival model

From even this cursory consideration of visual perspective it is possible to draw some elements that will help us construct a model of perspective and to understand the proper use of this metaphor in ethics.

First, there are the *sources* of, or input to, the standpoint, by which I shall mean those factors that determine how things will look to a percipient situated at that standpoint. Among these are the observer's distances from the objects viewed, the face each object presents to her, and the angle of her vision with respect to them. We can expand these sources, if we wish, to include other factors that affect how things look to her, for example, the amount of ambient light, the extent to which the faces presented are shadowed, and the presence or absence of mists or other obstacles to vision.

Second, there is what I shall call the *content* of the standpoint, by which I shall mean the view one gets from that standpoint, how things look from there. This will include such facts as whether a cup's rim looks round or ovoid, and whether railroad tracks appear parallel or convergent.

Third, there are the *objective judgments* an observer makes that are based, in part, at least, on her observations. The judgments to which I refer are objective in that they are about how the object is (whether, for example, the cup's rim is round), not about how it appears to the subject observing it. The sensible observer, of course, will rely on her own observations but will always modulate them with additional information gathered about others' (or her own earlier or later) observations as well as with information about visual distortions her standpoint's sources are likely to have caused.

We can draw three lessons pertinent to our concerns from this brief consideration of visual perspective. First, the fact that when we examine a certain field of inquiry, we encounter therein an extramental and extrapersonal order does not exclude the existence and legitimacy of perspectival variation within that area. We can give what I call a realistic interpretation of perspective, that is, an understanding of perspective that embeds it within a general theory that the things on which there are various perspectives themselves inhabit a single universe and are themselves "extramental" in the sense we introduced earlier.[25]

Against the claims of the cultural relativists, then, we can accept Banner's first thesis, that ethics (like visual perception) involves an extramental order (B1), while we reject his second thesis, that perspective has no appropriate place in such a realm (B2), thus allowing for the existence and legitimacy of differing perspectives in ethics, even differing ethnic perspectives in ethics. This moves us closer to answering the second of our initial questions; that is, it affords some understanding of how it may be possible for there to be ethnic perspectives on normative issues.

Second, even as in the case of visual perception we can approach a better understanding of *how something objectively is* by accumulating and reflecting on data about how it appears to people from different standpoints, so too in ethics we may be able to come to a better understanding of *how things objectively ought to be* by similarly accumulating and reflecting on information about the value judgments people make from different moral points of view.

Thus, we to begin to answer another of our initial questions, the third one concerning the good to be derived from such a perspective. We begin to see the good of differing ethical perspectives once we are aware that gathering and thinking about them better enables us to approach the truth in morals. It is in part by pondering the fact that the cup's rim looks ovoid when viewed from an angle but round when viewed from directly above that we are able to correct the distorted view of things inherent in a single, limited perspective. So, too, attention to the differing perspectives that African-Americans have on issues in medical ethics may be the much needed corrective to the distorted view we have, if we attend only to the opinions of medical and medical-ethics professionals (whose numbers will almost assuredly be disproportionately white, educated, and wealthy).

Third, we now have a model for the kinds of changes a difference in perspective can afford. In visual perception, such changes may include the following: (1) making objects look larger or smaller relative to one another; (2) bringing some objects to the foreground while others recede into the background; (3) altering an object's apparent contours; (4) allowing us to see sides of the object previously hidden from us, (5) permitting us to examine certain details heretofore unnoticed, while setting aside others that had earlier monopolized our attention; and (6) revealing to us patterns that are invisible from other angles.

Perspectives in ethics

We should expect corresponding transformations in, and corrections to, our view of moral issues once we take different ethical perspectives more seriously. As Cheryl Sanders writes about African-American and European-American perspectives, "both perspectives are operating within one moral universe and not two, and . . . each brings a valid critique to bear upon the other."[26]

This model of the sources of, content in, and judgments about ideas based on perspective, borrowed from our treatment of visual perception, furnishes us with a glimpse of an answer to the first of our questions: what is it for a position on ethical issues to reflect or involve an ethnic perspective? It is, however, only the barest glimpse. Plainly, there can be differing *ideological* perspectives on issues in applied ethics, for to take such a perspective is to approach the issue from an intellectual (and emotional) position shaped by, among other things, the values, principles, conceptions of human beings and their place in the world, and other values that define the ideology. Thus, there is no problem in supposing that there are, for example, meaningfully, and even distinctively, Marxist or *laissez faire* perspectives on some issues in health care. For similar reasons, it should be obvious that there can be differing *religious* perspectives on such issues. To take, for example, an Islamic perspective on these matters is to approach them from an initial position both constrained and partially formed by the normative and faith commitments constitutive of Islam and, perhaps, by certain other elements (for example, narratives) in that tradition.

To affirm all this is not to say that we should expect there to be a *single* Marxist (or Islamic) perspective. The commitments internal to an ideology or a religious denomination will be part of the approach that committed inquirers will adopt on the normative issues they investigate and should serve to constrain the kinds of moral view they will accept. These commitments, however, will not be the only factors informing their inquiry and, even if these commitments remain *exactly* the same across all inquirers committed to a certain credo or ideology (which is unlikely, since interpretations vary widely even of texts whose authority within the group is unquestioned), other factors are sure to vary among these similarly committed inquirers and these variations will suffice to constitute different perspectives even *within* the religious or ideological group. Thus, the proper question is never "What is *the* Marxist (or Islamic) perspective on these issues?" but some more complicated one such as, "When can an inquiry or position be properly said to reflect a Marxist (or Islamic) perspective?"

It is not so easy to say just how we ought to understand the concept of an *ethnic* perspective on such matters. Membership in a certain ethnic group cannot be defined in terms of an individual's values, principles, or other commitments. Sometimes partisans attempt something similar, insisting that a certain individual is not really a member of the ethnic group because she does not have the "right" ideas, but these efforts merely substitute some stipulated group "essence" for membership criteria that in reality are matters of ancestry, geography, pigmentation.[27]

Frantz Fanon protests against what he sees as Sartre's effort to establish an "essence" of being black, complaining that it goes against the grain of the existentialist doctrine that it is the task of the individual to determine the meaning of her own life.

> And so [for Sartre] it is not I who make a meaning for myself, but it is the meaning that was already there, pre-existing, waiting for me. . . . The black consciousness is held out as an absolute density, as filled with itself . . . Jean-Paul Sartre, in this work, has destroyed black zeal.[28]

Some black writers have recently expressed dissatisfaction with related efforts, all too frequently encountered, to read people out of the race on the basis of their political views, aesthetic tastes, or other attitudes.[29]

The case of ideological and religious perspectives does, I think, offer some guidance to our efforts to understand ethnic perspectives, and we shall return to that somewhat later. At this point, however, I will conclude this section by observing that, however we end up construing the concept of an ethnic perspective in applied ethics, if even the explicitly valuative components of a particular ideology or religious faith are normally insufficient strictly to determine a single perspective for all adherents, then surely we can expect that there will be no *single* African-American perspective on such issues. This is all the more obvious when we take into account that some African-Americans will themselves have ideological or religious commitments that must, by their nature, help shape the perspective from which those individuals view normative issues.

COMMUNITARIAN PERSPECTIVALISM, THE THIRD RESPONSE

The last line of response to Banner's challenge denies all three of that challenge's constituent theses, but it serves our purpose to concentrate on its denial of the third thesis, the claim that all humans make up only a single moral community, which community then provides its members a single rational and humane perspective from which they are to assess issues in applied ethics (B3). This thesis is dubious on its face. A community, properly speaking, is a group of people united in joint pursuit of shared goals, and it is not the case that all mankind stands so united. Some Western philosophers have lately seen in communities, so conceived and extending over generations, the source of moral values.[30] Like the cultural relativists, they accept a relativity thesis holding that moral judgments and practices are always the judgments and practices *of some group*, as well as a diversity thesis holding that traditions change over time and from place to place.[31]

On the communitarian's view, as in relativism, a person's moral judgments and life are pervaded by cultural perspective, and by ethnic and racial perspective insofar as ethnicity or race is tied to a determinate cultural tradition. Their view is like that of a recent poet who writes,

> *Whatever you have to say, leave*
> *the roots on, let them*
> *dangle*
> *And the dirt*
> > *Just to make clear*
> > *where they come from.*[32]

The communitarian's position is that in morals, at least, we have no choice but to "leave the roots on" our judgments, for they spring from and have meaning only within a cultural tradition. According to communitarianism's most prominent spokesperson, when we attempt to cut them off from the form of life and the socially-accepted standards in which they arose, we can no longer adjudicate between competing moral claims and our moral discourse descends into a sort of "emotivism," in which each side puts forward what appears to be a statement of fact about how things really are or ought to be but in fact is merely an expression of private feelings lacking any external standard of justification.[33]

Against Banner, communitarians contend that there is no one "rational and humane perspective" open to all humankind, for they follow Hegel in insisting that "rationality" and "humanity" are concepts too thin and insubstantial to do the necessary work of fixing an objective set of determinate values and principles. Rather, in the moral sphere, they are closer to the position Banner disapprovingly quotes from de Maistre; that is, people judge and act not as the Enlightenment's abstract "Man," but as "Frenchmen, Italians, or Russians," or, as modern communitarians might update de Maistre to add, as Frenchwomen, Yoruba, Navajo, Hmong, or African-American.[34]

Appraising cultural traditions

The communitarian, at least of the sort in which I am here interested, differentiates her position from that of the cultural relativist by her insistence that there are rational and objective grounds on which to evaluate elements from conflicting traditions. While she rejects the Cartesian dream that we can simply think ourselves free of the bonds of culture, she accepts the importance of constantly expanding and informing her perspective by bringing into it information about how things are seen and felt from other perspectives. The communitarian lacks the Cartesian confidence that we can easily slip the intellectual constraints culture imposes on us, but she also denies the assumption that cultural inheritance is primarily a hindrance to the free flight of reason; she sees it instead as a solid and secure base camp from which to make her expeditions into the unfamiliar. Nonetheless, despite her neo-Hegelian exaltation of culture and tradition, the communitarian accepts a critical perspective as an ideal we can approach asymptotically. Thus, even if it is still recognizably the perspective of some cultural group, it will have undergone and been altered by a process of critical engagement with challenges posed both from within the tradition (challenges of consistency) and from outside it.[35]

The communitarian maintains that any healthy, growing, and self-renewing cultural tradition continually subjects itself to various

forms of criticism. First, it seeks greater internal consistency of commitment and consistency in conforming practice to professed ideals.
Second, it strives to be open to learn from and be influenced by other
traditions and, to that end, encourages its adherents to expose their
minds to other possibilities. Third, it has enough flexibility to adjust
to changing circumstances and to offer guidance beyond familiar and
predictable situations. Fourth, it demands that its adherents subject
opposed traditions to the same tests of consistency and adaptability.

Indeed, communitarians recognize that, on their view, there can
be no nonrelativized *moral* standard by which to judge cultures, no
timeless and neutral moral rank-ordering. Hence, they place great
emphasis precisely on such *contextual* superiority. A given cultural
tradition demonstrates a kind of contextual superiority over a differing tradition when, for example, it passes a test of internal self-consistency while the latter tradition fails a corresponding test, or when it
solves, in a way that even those within the second tradition can recognize as superior to their own tradition's efforts, problems that are
recognized within the latter. For the communitarian, there can be no
transcendental deduction proving that this tradition is the only rational way of organizing a group's moral life, nor any single test showing that it is better than every possible (or even every actual)
alternative. It may even be that a given tradition's ability to pass tests
for self-consistency (and other tests) which other traditions fail,
thereby demonstrating its superiority over those other traditions on a
case-by-case basis, is the best for which its adherents can reasonably
hope. And they probably won't even get that.

I suspect that some of the arguments marshalled earlier against
cultural relativism will also work against communitarianism, for they
were directed primarily against the relativists' relativity and diversity
theses, to which communitarians are also committed.[36] I won't, however, pursue those misgivings here. My point in this section has
merely been to sketch a third line of response, one less strongly realistic than the line proceeding from the analogy with visual perception,
but a line somewhat more plausible and appealing than most versions
of the cultural relativism we discussed in the earlier part of this paper.
Some communitarians may also hold the belief that while there is no
acultural access to a transcendent order of moral truth, there are yet
facts to which any account of morality must ultimately answer—facts
about human beings, their nature and needs, their origins and
destiny—and they may join to that belief the further hope that this
process of cultural criticism, testing, and winnowing may in the end

bequeath to us a perspective on our moral life that is not only newer and more comprehensive but also truly adequate to those facts.

WHERE WE STAND, ASSESSING OUR RESPONSES

The preceding considerations, if they have been at all successful, show that those who wish to identify, develop, or articulate African-American perspectives on issues in biomedical ethics have at least options in attempting to make sense of their project. It may be useful to summarize where we stand. For the reasons given above, and for others as well, I am skeptical about the cultural relativists' position, and I see no good reason to follow them in denying the thesis that the moral order is in some important senses genuinely extramental (B1).

In my judgment, however, this thesis should be rejected because the realist interpretation of perspectives (according to which they are confined to the realm of appearances) is well-grounded and intuitively appealing. Some will object that on such a view perspectives are unimportant, but I have tried to show why that is not so. The realist can concede that while there is an order of reality beyond any one perspective (perhaps even beyond *all* perspectives), understanding and learning from the various perspectives may be an important means of access to that order. The realist may even consistently say that one's perspective is the necessary starting point in the ascent to objective truth. Sanders makes a similar claim about theology: "All theologies have a contextual point of departure and may be rooted in the particularities of human experience, even if their ultimate conclusions point toward universal revelation."[37] It is difficult for me to see how a perspective could have greater importance than the importance ceded in recognizing it as a significant, perhaps even a necessary, access to objective truth.

Banner's third thesis maintains that all humankind is united in a single moral community sharing a single rational perspective (B3). This strikes me as extravagant and seems wrongheaded unless we employ a concept of community so broad as to render the statement empty. Moreover, the communitarians have a lesson to teach about the need to critique and transcend even the traditions in which we feel at home, a point to which we shall return later. Despite my sympathy for some elements in the communitarians' view and for their rejection of B3, I have serious misgivings about their line of response to Banner's challenge. That response, as I mentioned, seems to me to share with cultural relativism certain crucial defects. My conclusion, then, is that the second line of response, with its realist interpretation of perspectives, is the most promising.

AFRICAN-AMERICAN ETHICAL PERSPECTIVES

As we remarked earlier, it is not obvious just how to answer the first of our initial questions: What is it to view a normative issue from an ethnic perspective? Our best strategy, I think, is to work from what we have already learned about visual perspective and about the meaning of viewing a normative issue from the perspective of a particular ideology or religious doctrine. Unlike being a Marxist or a Muslim, being an African-American does not consist in, or even entail, being committed to any set of values, principles, or other beliefs. There may, of course, be certain opinions or feelings we think it somehow suitable for an African-American to have, and we may even be right to think that, but having them is never a necessary condition for belonging to the ethnic group.[38] It follows that taking an African-American perspective on a normative issue cannot consist in viewing it from a standpoint partially shaped by the commitments constitutive of being African-American. In principle, there are and can be no such constituent commitments.[39]

Developing the sources

Similarly, we need to avoid the attempt to ground African-American perspectives in biological or stereotypical materials. Dinesh D'Souza worries that "unless we are willing to sanction the idea of natural [that is, biological] difference between races—seemingly a racist idea—it is pointless and possibly dangerous to sanction the validity of 'white' and 'black' perspectives, any more than we can approve the old Nazi notion of 'Jewish science.'" Similarly, he warns against the example of one scholar who upholds fallacious argument, incivility, and sexist arrogance as elements of black "culture."[40] There is cause for concern here.

Psychologist Janet Helms summarizes the work of a dozen social scientists from the 1970s and 1980s, each of whom claims to be able to assign a black person to a "typological" category or a psychological developmental stage. For example, one typological model arranges us into "Coloreds," who are said to evaluate themselves "by White standards," "Negroes," who don't know how they feel about themselves or about white people; and "Blacks," who, we find out, are "no longer ashamed of African racial characteristics." One of the developmental models plots an individual's possible psychological ascent through stages from an "Identification with Oppressed People" to a culminating stage called "Affirmation of Blackness."[41]

Helms introduces the term "negriscence" for "the developmental process by which a person 'becomes Black'" by progressively moving away "from least healthy, White-defined stages of identity." She claims to be able to measure this movement with the help of an "instrument" she devised with Thomas A. Parham. This "instrument," called the "Black Racial Identity Attitude Scale" measures respondents according to how much they agree with such statements as "The most important thing about me is that I am Black" and "I frequently confront the system and the man." (The comparable scale for white people asks, interestingly enough, for feelings about more ambivalent or even wistful statements—e.g., "I hardly think about what race I am" and "I wish I had a black friend.") Those selected to answer the questionnaire are deceived about its true name, and told only that it measures "social and political attitudes." They are also told that no answers are "right or wrong," but not told that they will be judged more or less black.[42] Helms's developmental model is a complicated one according to which a person's racial identity comprises three types of identification: "ascribed identity," which concerns one's "deliberate affiliation or commitment to a racial group"; "personal identity," which concerns her "feelings and attitudes about [her]self"; and "reference group-identity, which concerns "the extent to which one uses particular racial groups . . . to guide one's feelings, thoughts, and behaviors." These "identities," in turn, are analyzed in relation to "worldviews," "sociocultural communicators," "foci," and so on.[43]

Unfortunately for our purposes, Helms's elaborate apparatus yields few specifics about what might be the content of an African-American ethical perspective, not even much about how and what most of us think about ethics. In discussing "worldviews," the most we hear is that another writer has claimed that Africans differ from Europeans in a tendency toward "groupness [sic] rather than individuality . . . cooperation rather than competition . . . [and] greater belief in 'survival of the tribe' rather than 'survival of the fittest'."[44] That is not much to go on.

There are other reasons to worry about this research. In Helms's own developmental model, and in every one of the others that she presents, the black person at the lowest psychological level, the one who is least healthy is variously described as one who "depends on White society for self-definition," "copes by imitating Whites," is "antagonistic to conversion to Blackness," "identifies with White culture," and so on. In contrast, those at higher levels are those who "internalize Black culture," achieve "pride in one's ethnicity," "abandon the White definition of self," and so on. Helms observes that a person who surveys this literature "cannot help but notice further striking similarities in stage content across the various models . . . [all of which] appeared in the literature around the same time."

Since the researchers were working independently of one another and studying populations in different cities, Helms reasons, "The similarity, then, is not so much with the models, but in the phenomena observed." This inference, however, is too hasty, for the similarity could stem from a bias shared by the researchers. I am not in a position to say whether this is true, but there are grounds for doubt. After all, the time when this research was being done and published coincided with or shortly followed the "Black Pride" movement, the publication of Frantz Fanon's Black Skin, White Masks (a work that must have had a powerful impact on black social scientists of the time), and growing disfavor with the "color-blind," integrationist program of the most prominent civil rights leaders of the 1950s and early 1960s. Indeed, the language of many of the researchers cited by Helms mirrors and may be drawn from the rhetoric and self-perception of the militants of the time.

In light of these facts, how do we know that the theorists of what Helms calls "negriscence" have not allowed political views to shape their conclusions about who and what is psychologically healthy? It is also unclear why this developmental process, even if real, should be considered a process of, in Helms's phrase, "becoming black." In some of the developmental models, including Helms's own, the highest stage is one in which the individual transcends racial hostility and reduction of the self to race. It seems likely that this would count as progress not only for black people but for anyone.

Helms's work lends itself to an illegitimate psychologizing of politics. I have heard one of her former students use it to dismiss Judge Clarence Thomas's views on affirmative action, attributing them to his undeveloped racial identity. This is merely an instance of what logicians call the "genetic fallacy," that is, of allowing speculations about what drives an individual to hold a certain belief do the work for the much harder task of examining the evidence available for and against the belief's truth. I disagree with neoconservative claims that preferential treatment breeds black self-doubt and white resentment, or unfairly victimizes innocent people. Still, the important questions are these political ones about the merits of preferential treatment. They cannot be replaced by questions about the psychological development or lack of development among their opponents or proponents.

Of course, Helms cannot be held responsible for every misuse of her theories, and it is to be hoped that she repudiates this one. Still, her own method of correlating an individual's "decision-making style" and "cognitive style" with her racial identity "attitude" is problematic in a related way. Her "Black Racial Identity Attitude Scale," asks the respondent whether, for example, she "feels very uncomfortable around Black people." If, however, Helms takes an affirmative answer to indicate little development in "negriscence," and correlates this with what are held to be white "cognitive styles" and "cultural attitudes," then the difficulty appears. For, suppose a person's political thinking incites her political opponents to use racial invective against her, and that this rhetoric succeeds in convincing other black people that she is an Uncle Tom and a race traitor. Then, she may understandably begin to feel "very uncomfortable" around them. For the psychologist to use this discomfort as an indicator of an undeveloped "racial identity attitude" is clearly illegitimate, because its cause is plainly political and interpersonal rather than psychological.[45]

Obviously, neither biological science nor the sort of social science that elevates stereotypical or dysfunctional behavior into "culture" can be adequate sources in our search to understand African-American outlooks. Yet we also know that African-Americans have typically undergone certain experiences, suffered from certain health afflictions, been under represented in the biomedical professions in comparison to white representation, and over represented among the poor and uneducated in comparison to white representation. Annette Dula has suggested that African-American perspectives on issues in bioethics are largely shaped by these differences in our experience of health care, an insight that assists our attempt to sketch an answer to our question.[46] We should add that other experiences will also matter here. Harley Flack and Edmund Pellegrino have written:

> Slavery, segregation, discrimination, poverty, and a disadvantaged position with respect to education, health, and medical care, sensitize African-Americans in specific ways [evoking from them] a more empathetic response to the social-ethical questions—justice in the distribution of resources, sensitivity to the vulnerability of the sick person, and a sense of responsibility for the poor and rejected members of society."[47]

The history and types of encounters African-Americans have frequently had with white Americans in various professions and institutions (governmental, corporate, and educational) will also influence the perspectives we are likely to take on questions about how health care professionals and institutions ought to behave.[48] Using the model we developed above, we can say that these experiences and history will serve as *sources* of the perspective with which we are concerned. We should not expect to uncover a slant that is either universal among us or peculiar to us. What we can hope for, however, is a variety of outlooks that are *meaningfully* African-American in that each is, in significant measure, shaped by experiences or activities that are characteristic of African-American people.

Prudence dictates that I leave it to those who are knowledgeable about, and skilled in using, health care statistics and the relevant histories (of African-Americans and American medicine) to depict this experience and to offer us guidance about its *content* and the objective ethical *judgments* it best supports. I will, however, offer a few suggestions here that may be of interest, though more as a type of content than as a guide to the actual content such perspectives may have.[49]

In visual perception, one's particular standpoint will affect how large things look, what shapes they seem to have, which of their sides and details are visible, and whether certain lines appear to meet. Using this analogy, we may expect that in ethics one's standpoint will influence such factors as how much weight is accorded some facts, how a problem is configured, what aspects of a problem are noticed, and whether lines of reasoning normally opposed to one another appear to converge on a common conclusion. Sanders has recently suggested that the "ethos" of African-Americans is "essentially holistic," while that of Americans of European descent is dualistic; inclusive, where the other is exclusive; communalistic, where the other is individualistic; spiritual, where the other is intellectual; theistic, where the other is agnostic or atheistic; improvisational in its approach, where the other is structured; and humanistic, where the other is materialistic.[50] Without doubt, more work needs to be done in sociology and history before we can know whether these claims are true, and more in philosophy before we can know how to understand the contrasts.[51]

Delineating the content

It is, as I have said, for other speakers or for future researchers to delineate in detail the common content or characteristic of any perspective on bioethical matters that is meaningfully African-American. I will, however, try to assist their efforts by offering first, and with considerable hesitation, a few very tentative suggestions about some features that might be characteristic of such a perspective, and then a few suggestions about how some practical issues might look from such a standpoint. My hope is, in that way, to stimulate discussion among those of you who have more knowledge about these matters than I can claim.

The characteristic content of a perspective that is shaped by certain typical aspects of African-American history and experience (especially, by our experience of health care systems, their institutions and personnel) will vary depending on which elements of that experience exert pressure, how strong that pressure is, what other factors in the individual's life may counteract these elements, how strong and of what type these opposed factors might be, and on much else besides. Despite the necessary uncertainty in these matters, it might help to clarify and illustrate this rather abstract analysis of perspective, if I hazard a few concrete surmises about its content, that is, about how things might look from an African-American perspective. I make no claim that these elements, individually or collectively, are exclusively or even distinctively African-American. Collectively, however, I think that they can comprise a perspective that is meaningfully African-American in the sense that it is shaped by our characteristic experiences. I should add at once that these surmises are based on no surveys and even the impressions on which they are based come from my own unrepresentative experience and inadequate amount of reading and reflection. Indeed, they probably better sketch the kinds of outlook I think it is sensible for us to have than the kinds we do have. Nonetheless, if I am to illustrate what I take a perspective in ethics to be, it is better that I give even a bad illustration than none at all. So, with those disclaimers and warnings on record, I will proceed to the task.

(1) Such a perspective is likely to be anti-majoritarian and anti-utilitarian. One obvious reason to be dissatisfied with majoritarianism is that African-Americans, as a minority group, have little to gain from majoritarian principles. A deeper and less obvious reason is that our experience as a minority has taught us how wrong and unjust the majority can be in the pursuit of its own interests. This heightened sense of justice impels one to direct resources in one's own or in the public's hands toward the neediest rather than to spread them out among the largest number. Most notably in the civil rights movement, but elsewhere besides, constraints on the majority are expressed in terms of individual rights, so rights should loom large from this vantage.

Majoritarian thinking is a type of maximization strategy and is often tied to the philosophical theory of direct utilitarianism, which directs agents to perform the action likely to have the best results.[52] This sort of theory has come under attack on many grounds but, even aside from explicit majoritarianism, some of its little-discussed features make utilitarianism especially unattractive to those concerned with minority rights. In an important essay, Robert M. Veatch has argued that a priority principle of the sort utilitarians favor, one assigning such scarce resources as donated organs to those likely to derive greatest medical benefit from them, will sometimes work in a predictable way to the disadvantage of African-Americans, even in the absence of racist discrimination.[53] There are several reasons. Those who are economically disadvantaged or acculturated into dysfunctional values and behavior patterns may be in worse shape (than the privileged) by the time transplantation is considered, because they may not be in the habit of frequent medical check-ups and healthful lifestyles. Moreover, mistrust and unfamiliarity with medical institutions may make them more unlikely to serve as donors, thus making donor-recipient matches less common. For right now at least, there is a further difficulty. Because African-Americans are harder to assign to a tissue type than others are, they are less likely to be identified as good (that is, as matching)—less likely, in other words, to be designated as ones in whom the transplanted organs will probably thrive.

Veatch emphasizes that his point is not restricted to racial minorities.

> There are many other groups that will lose if a policy is in place allocating solely on the basis of years of life expected from the graft. Women have greater incidence of antibodies than men, making it harder to find organs; recipients of blood group O are harder to match. Older persons have statistically fewer years of life added with a transplant. A good utilitarian who is using years of life added per organ transplanted as the criterion of utility will purposely accept an allocation formula giving low probabilities of transplanting these groups. Someone committed to a theory of justice . . . will want to adjust the allocation formula so as to give members of these groups a fair shot.[54]

In repudiating utilitarianism, I think those whose ethical perspective is meaningfully informed by characteristically African-American experiences may also be inclined to reject the doctrine that the end justifies the means. In deciding what to do, it is always pertinent to look to the quality of one's action and the way in which it relates the agent to another. It is said that when Justice William O. Douglas asked Justice Thurgood Marshall to join him in a decision declaring racial discrimination against white people unconstitutional, Marshall replied: "You guys have been practicing discrimination for years. Now it's our turn." If the story is true, Marshall was presumably being facetious, and surely most African-Americans would, like me, deny that white people who lose positions owing to affirmative action programs are victims of racial discrimination. Still, a remark like Marshall's, if meant to be serious, offends the heightened sense of justice we can expect of those injured by discrimination.

It might be thought that for African-Americans to recognize that there are means even the noblest ends cannot justify, also requires them to reject the famous liberationist slogan of Malcolm X: "By any means necessary." This thought, however, is not entirely correct. The maxim that one can do anything "necessary" to achieve one's end, even the best end, is surely one that people with any real understanding of justice will find repugnant, and one from which Malcolm X ought more clearly to have distanced himself. Still, I doubt that it was that maxim that he had in mind. The social context in which the remark gained notoriety was a criticism of the pacifist doctrine of nonviolence according to which nonviolence is praised not only as an effective strategy for liberation but as the only morally acceptable one—the debate, still with us, between Malcolm and Martin Luther King, Jr. That was also its oratorical context, as one his last speeches indicates.

In that address, he uses the phrase several times, saying, for example, "Our objective is complete freedom, complete justice, complete equality, by any means necessary." Just before he stressed that black people should be willing to kill such people as the racist thugs who had brutalized voting rights activist Fannie Lou Hamer, who shared the platform on that occasion, Malcolm X stressed the importance of their ability to vote for it, "And by being registered [on voting lists] as independents, it means we can do whatever is necessary, wherever it's necessary, and whenever the time comes. Do you understand?" The peroration of that speech emphasizes that his point was simply the moral permissibility of violence against unjust aggressors. "I don't accept any nonviolent liberals. This doesn't mean you have to be violent. But it does mean you can't be nonviolent."[55] His point was to rebut those who opposed all violence in liberation struggles as a matter of principle. He thus spoke up for the moral permissibility and propriety of violence directed against aggressors when necessary for the defense of self and others, without in fact saying that violence was necessary. For Malcolm X to say this at a time when there was reason to fear that elite praise for the pacificist nonviolence of King and others might delegitimize self-defense among black people, was, in retrospect, an act of courage and a defense of what was surely a moral position traditional in the West.

(2) It should prove anti-situationist. Sanders may be correct that it is part of our ethos to favor improvisational methods over structured. Nonetheless, African-Americans have much to fear from health-care decisions that flow, not from established and publicized policies that have been defended before the public and interest groups, but from some individual's or group's seat-of-the-pants "judgment" about whether, for example, a patient's life is sufficiently worthwhile to warrant resuscitation. Such decision makers are likely to have little in common in terms of personal experiences, social or economic stratum, interests, tastes, or educational level with the African-Americans at their mercy. The patient, it seems, should be entitled to the protection of announced and codified procedures.

(3) For the same reasons, such a perspective will be inclined to *distrust* the "ethics of trust" that some physicians espouse.[56] Professional degrees earned in, and under the ethical norms of, institutions that themselves have demonstrated no great sensitivity to African-Americans and their needs will appear to be a poor basis for trust, when it is the patient's very health and life that are being entrusted to the professional's tender mercies. The African-American is entitled to a certain skepticism, if not cynicism, about the basis for this trust, especially if it seems to involve no demonstration of concern for us.

This skepticism can literally be a matter of life and death if physicians are empowered to advise and assist in the termination not only of a patient's treatment but of her life as well, as legislation in Washington state recently proposed. When a person, already poor and sick, has also had her sense of self-worth eroded by experience as the object of racist attitudes and practices, she needs to be assured that her life is important and that others value her, in spite of the burdens that caring for her may impose on them. Instead, it is suggested that medical personnel should present themselves to this desperate, needy soul and offer their services to help speed her down the path that illness has already marked for her. Perhaps even more troubling is the current trend to entrust decisions about whether to sustain the life of the incompetent ill to already burdened family members, despite the obvious and inherent conflict of interest. In such cases, the idea presented as a right to self-determination reveals itself as a ticket to self-extermination.[57]

(4) Although Robert Murray thinks, perhaps correctly, that autonomy may not figure as prominently in African-American moral thinking as it does in European-American thought; still, the patient should

be regarded as the one with the decision to make.[58] Only such empowerment frees her from dangerous total dependence on those who may neither understand nor genuinely sympathize with her. These dangers may be less acute when the health care providers are themselves African-Americans, but it remains difficult to see how the patient wins real freedom or justice if control over her life is wrested from white professionals or bureaucrats only to be thrown to black ones.[59]

(5) Such a perspective is likely to prove sympathetic to, but unromantic about, families. Black families in America seldom fit the "Father Knows Best" model. It is, I suspect, more common among African-American families than among European-American families that a grandparent, an aunt, an uncle will play a significant part of the role usually assigned to the mother or father in that model. I don't think we should accept that as merely a neutral fact, let alone exalt it as a bold and innovative arrangement for the family, a testament to our creativity in social structures. Research on the "feminization" and juvenilization of poverty indicate that this is a breakdown of the family, not its reinforcement, and a tragedy of the first order, surely one of the gravest in our lives today.

Indeed, I would think this arrangement a bad thing even apart from its economic consequences. But the alarming statistics on poverty and impairment among children in single-parent families makes it clear even to those who are reluctant to acknowledge it that children should live with their parents, and their parents should live together, married, for life. Nevertheless, it is a fact that our families are often both less inclusive (because of absent parents, usually fathers) and more inclusive (because of the greater role played by grandparents, aunts or uncles) than the traditional picture. The fact has implications. On the one hand, it indicates that forces which would further erode family life or parental authority must be strenuously resisted. Provisions for family involvement (for example, parental consent or notification) must be flexible enough to meet the situation of families in which a grandparent, or aunt, or other surrogate, is acting in the role of parent. On the other hand, we should not assume that family members, even parents, always have the best interests of the family at heart. It would be lovely and romantic were that always true, but it is not.

From such a perspective, I think, policies strengthening parental authority, especially over the behavior of teenagers in those areas in which they are least likely to act responsibly, will seem on the whole desirable. In contrast, policies giving a family member direct and solitary control over the life and health of another will seem unwise and dependent on romantic assumptions about the nobility of kinsfolk. Those who live in neighborhoods populated by "boarder babies" and children infected with AIDS induced by parental drug-abuse should know that we cannot simply assume that parents will act in their children's best interest.[60]

(6) Such a perspective, in part because it is *not* bound to scientism, is likely to be informed by religious faith. While there have been important African-American scientists, engineers, technologists, and inventors, we are, I suspect, less inclined to claim advances in these fields as our distinctive achievement, and therefore less tempted by the epistemology of scientism, according to which position all knowledge and even all rational belief must be experimentally testable. Sensible people find this epistemology absurd on its face, and logical positivism, the major effort to give it philosophical articulation, failed badly, sometimes falling victim to self-referential incoherence. (The verificationists' claim, that the meaning of a statement is the means used to verify it, is, of course, the most celebrated case of this incoherence.) Nonetheless, it continues to exert strong influence in the Western world on academics, policy-makers, and lawyers.

African-Americans are not at all immune to such thinking, but for us it holds out less hope for ratifying our place in the world. We are, as a consequence, less apt to worry about whether or not our beliefs and behavior are "rational" by some stringent scientistic standard. (Such a standard is literally pseudo-scientific in that it imitates science, falls short of the mark, and yet still pretends to be scientific.) This assertion has implications for political morality, to which we will turn shortly, but first we should note a different result.

Rejecting scientism does not require, either logically or psychologically, adopting any religious belief. Nevertheless, this rejection does remove or lessen one powerful hindrance to such faith. Among African-Americans, religious commitment, especially forms of Protestant Christianity, has traditionally played an important role in community life. Perhaps for that reason, even African-American intellectuals and academics seem, to me, to be more unapologetically religious than is common among white intellectuals and academics. We should expect religion, therefore, to be a powerful influence shaping the perspective of most African-Americans.

(7) If African-Americans are characteristically less anxious about whether their beliefs and behavior meet some exceptionally elevated and inappropriate standard of rationality and testability, then modern neutralist political morality may also seem less appealing from our point of view. That should be true, at least, to the extent that political doctrine relies on the (doubtful) claim that the state (a) is

justified in acting on determinate principles of social justice because some such principles can be shown to meet a high standard of rationality, and (b) is not justified in acting from any determinate conception of what kind of life is good for people because no such conception can be shown to meet these standards.

Rejecting neutralist political theory can have important implications for public health policy, since the discussion of such policy is sometimes short-circuited by appeal to neutralist theory. I will illustrate that in the next part of this section, when I turn to the question of what options in medical ethics might seem morally attractive or unattractive from a standpoint at least partially shaped by these factors.

Applying moral judgments

It is unclear to me that these characteristics of an African-American perspective, even in conjunction with other plausible candidates, will suffice strictly to afford determinate answers to complex issues in biomedical ethics. We will probably settle not only for a variety of African-American perspectives, but also for a variety of conflicting moral conclusions. Still, the characteristics tentatively suggested in the previous section do shape one's standpoint in such a way that certain options appear morally attractive and others morally inadequate. It may be useful to mention a few options of these kinds and to try, in a cursory way, to link their disposition to some of the characteristics mentioned above.

My discussion will do little more than speculate about general conclusions, omitting the qualifications, distinctions, and responses to objections that lend moral arguments philosophical interest. Others will probably want to concentrate on issues in distributive justice such as those raised by Oregon's recent plans to restrain Medicaid funding or Britain's age-based restrictions on who may be dialyzed. Leaving those matters to people with better information and firmer convictions, my speculative comments will be on other topics. We won't agree here but, if nothing else, at least I will have illustrated my point that there are many perspectives among us, perspectives shaped not only by our reactions to shared experiences, but also by religious or ideological convictions and episodes in our private or family lives.

(1) Because of our hesitation to entrust control over life and death to physicians or family members, those considering mercy-killing and abortion from these points of view will incline to find them morally unacceptable. Other characteristics serve to reinforce this view. Once

someone's mind is freed from the constraints of secularism, she is less likely to feel confident she knows just when someone's life has stopped being worth living in such a way that justifies us in pursuing her death. Indeed, she may think that the lives of suffering, disabled, or unconscious people are a good deal more enviable and valuable than are those of healthy people frittering away their lives on worldly thrills. But as she does not feel justified in putting the latter out of their pleasures, she will see even less justification for putting the former out of their misery.

Again, a heightened sense of justice that drives her to give priority to bringing even small incremental benefits to the neediest should dispose her against speeding the death of the sickest, the most disabled, the most defenseless, especially those not yet born.

Similarly, concern for the next generation of African-Americans should color her view of abortion policies that at present allow for the termination (with prejudice, as they say in another context) of more than one in three pregnancies among black females.[61] So must her reflection on the incentive and the message sent by policies whereby the state will defray most of the cost of killing the developing or potential child *in utero* but will absorb only a small fraction of the cost of supporting the child after birth. The discussion has become obscured by the reluctance of proponents of cheap, quick, and easy abortion to speak forthrightly. Their punctilious insistence on using such codewords as "choice" and "reproductive freedom," which divert public attention from the serious questions: what is being chosen? under what circumstances? as against what alternatives? and with what consequences? The rhetoric of "choice" should have less power to mesmerize minds attuned to how little choice the needy, the desperate, and the immature may feel themselves to have when confronted with such options. This problem is aggravated, of course, when self-proclaimed proponents of "choice" impede efforts to insure the integrity of choice by requiring that these painful decisions be made only after deliberation, with full information about side-effects and alternative procedures, and (in the case of minors) in consultation with guardians.

Sensitivity to the history of the eugenics movement's attacks on black people should also incline more thoughtful and sensitive African-Americans against the pro-choice and pro-abortion movements to the extent that these movements begin to revive the rhetoric of the eugenicist.[62]

(2) Someone whose ethical standpoint is characterized by the features we mentioned above should, I think, also be disposed to condemn proposals to distribute clean needles to drug abusers and

recent plans such as the ones made in New York City and in Maryland to distribute condoms free of charge to high school students in their school clinics. She will, at least, be disposed to reject such plans insofar as their support is supposed to derive from neutralist theories of political morality.

Suppose someone insists that the promotion and allocation of health care is one of the benefits of rationally-justified determinate principles of distributive justice. Therefore, these principles militate in favor of wide, free distribution of sterile needles and prophylactics and in favor of mass-media instruction in and promotion of their use. When it is objected that such policies undermine efforts of parents and churches to inculcate virtues of self-restraint, the neutralist can reply that she needn't prove any case against the value of these virtues.

Rather, according to her, the mere fact that there is widespread dispute among reasonable people about this conception of the good life or that a person could reasonably reject the principle enjoining the state to act so as to undermine self-restraint itself demonstrates that the objection has failed to give a reason from which the state could legitimately act in rejecting the proposals. For it could not properly repudiate the policy out of a concern to promote self-restraint among its citizens without showing illicit partiality for some conceptions of the good life over others. A perspective that rejects neutralist political theory, however, is free to view self-restraint as just one important good among many the state should be fostering.

Add to this the preference for support of parental authority and the need unambiguously to inculcate attitudes in which cheap thrills are set aside in favor of personal health and achievement. Drug abusers need to acquire the sort of concern for their health that might lead them to change their lives. To focus instead on getting them to change their needles and to do so in the name of health is apt only to confuse them. (I know it confuses me.) Similarly, teenagers desperately need help building the sort of character that will enable them to subordinate and restrict sexual pleasure and desire to the serious and lasting commitments that enhance the chances for stable marriage. The single-minded rush to prevent AIDS without addressing the deeper problems involved in habitual drug use and promiscuous sexual behavior will, I think, appear unattractive from a point of view informed by these concerns.

(3) A person with such a perspective who has also experienced being among the neediest will look askance at the tendency to make availability to health care contingent on the individual's ability to pay. The plight of the uninsured and the underinsured is dispropor-

tionally the plight of African-Americans, and decency requires that a person's medical needs not go unattended because he or she is also financially needy. A delivery system that permits the one disadvantage to exacerbate the other will be difficult to justify in any ethical perspective, especially one in which special attention is paid to questions of justice and minority interests.

Similarly, the moral legitimacy of initiatives, such as that recently taken in Oregon, designed to define and limit the state's obligation to pay for the health requirements of the impoverished, will face a stiff challenge. From an ethical perspective sensitized to the needs of the "invisible" and the "forgotten," it will be hard to see how it can be licit to save the money of the better-off by cutting back efforts to preserve the life or restore the health of the worst-off.

LOOKING AHEAD, ADMONITIONS, REFORMS, AND REVISIONS

We have now examined the questions of what an African-American perspective on bioethics is, and how things can look from such a standpoint. We have investigated how such a perspective may be possible, and what good it might be. But the fourth of our initial questions remains: What are some of the dangers and limitations that might lurk in identifying and attending to such a standpoint?

Some of what we have already said should prove helpful here, but I also want to draw on the work of Cheryl Sanders, who offers important insights. As we said above, part of the value of heeding neglected points of view is that doing so can help us correct for distortions in our earlier view. It can also help us rectify things we have done wrongly because of those distortions. Thus one danger is that we shall become so involved in merely articulating this perspective and in making it our own that we won't bring its insights to bear in correcting other standpoints and in formulating a critique of social practice.

Thus, according to Sanders, "the idea of a uniquely black ethic" is problematic if it does not "transcend its particularity at some points in order to bring critical commentary to bear on the society at large."[63] She eloquently reminds us that such a perspective "is ultimately a human perspective; a concrete, particular witness to universal truth. . . . This ethos should not merely be regarded as an interesting minority perspective or contribution, but rather should be in a position to inform the shape and content of the whole discourse."[64] We must, then, guard against the danger, a danger lurking within Alain Locke's blithe espousal of social reciprocity and tolerance, that leads us to adopt a possessive attitude. Once scholars have identified, articulated, and explained the components of an African-American ethical standpoint, we risk using it only for ourselves, having recourse to it when *we* need to make a decision or understand a problem, but failing to bring its insights to the labor involved in correcting the distortions in other standpoints.

This process of correction is a two-way street, however, and that fact exposes a second danger, one to which the communitarians should have alerted us. Again, Sanders put the point powerfully when she wrote of both the African-American and the European-American points of view: "each brings a valid critique to bear on the other. Both must be subjected to scrutiny by similar standards—it is as wrong to romanticize African-American culture as it is to overlook the racism that is endemic to Euro-American culture."[65] If this perspective is really to be part of a healthy and vital tradition, it must itself be opened to revision and improvement under the influence of insights gleaned from other perspectives and from reflection on our needs and experience. It is dangerous in a second way to treat it as sacrosanct, beyond improvement.

In this final section, I wish to anticipate the next stage, offering some remarks on how, I think, certain elements among the experiences and changed environment of African-Americans *ought* to affect our outlook so as to give greater emphasis to some values and de-emphasize others, and to alter the way we see ourselves, our communities, our culture, and that divided condition which the hyphen in the term "African-American" bridges so inadequately. These remarks are merely programmatic and intended to stimulate deeper investigation.

Pluralism over solidarity.

We cannot have both pluralism and solidarity, and we have already argued that any individual's standpoint will be shaped by a multiplicity of factors. The factors we suggested as influential in shaping distinctively African-American standpoints are insufficient either to define the standpoint in detail or to determine just what moral options are to be selected. It follows that there may well be diversity in our viewpoints and in our views. If uniformity of thought is not compelled by the characteristics that shape authentically African-American standpoints, then either we must ensure it by pressure (psychological or otherwise) or abandon it. The former course is morally and politically repugnant. Some recent black writers have protested these demands for conformity. As Stanley Crouch writes (a bit too caustically for my taste), "Varieties of speech rhythm, diction, accent, taste, and style are fine for white people, but [according to some black people] there must be a psychological and spiritual tub of tar a Negro should sit in each morning before facing the white day."[66]

Leonard Harris has contrasted the interest of most American philosophers to downplay or escape cultural influence (an interest that has characterized Western philosophy since Descartes), with some African-American philosophers' concern to emphasize and recapture cultural ties.[67] This concern is best seen, however, as a response to denials of the validity of black peoples' cultures. Once we are psychologically able to take the validity of our cultures for granted, our cultures, like those of others, can serve their proper role as starting points, not destinations, for the personal journeys of individuals.[68]

Even Mao Tse-Tung, that despicable oppressor whose prose the Black Panthers pretended to admire, professed an interest in letting a thousand flowers bloom.[69] (It must be admitted that his spiritual and political successors' penchant for mob rule [the Cultural Revolution] and mass extinction [Tiananmen Square] calls into doubt the sincerity of this expressed wish.) That idea still seems too extreme to some African-Americans who fancy themselves revolutionaries.[70]

Transvaluating individualism

This naturally follows from the preceding point. Shelby Steele has attacked those who, viewing "blacks as a racial monolith, a singular people with a common experience of oppression," decided that "differences within the race, no matter how ineradicable had to be minimized."[71] So conceived, "the black identity censors individuality by enforcing a rigid 'party line.'"[72] Once that party line, that psychological conformity, is abandoned, we may free ourselves from the narrow view in which "individualism is seen as selfishness and opportunism," as Charles Johnson writes.[73] Of course, that sort of individualism is to be discouraged. But, as Steele stresses, there can be no economic or social advancement of the race, once legal barriers are lowered, except insofar as individuals excel. True, those individuals shouldn't be selfish, as no one should be selfish. But they must see the possibilities and opportunities they have as ones they must take advantage of in virtue of what is special and different about them, not as what is shared. In that way we may begin to free ourselves and our children from what Charles Johnson calls the "pre-individualistic" phase of black thought and identity.[74]

It is also worth remembering that the great injustices inflicted on *black* people were inflicted on black *people*; it is individuals who suffer, who aspire to achieve, who have needs and rights. It is well and good to urge that an enhanced regard for the African-American communities' achievements be a part of the self-image of each of us, but the image of which these are part is an image of the individual's *self*.[75] "Talk of *the* Afro-American experience treats the complex worlds of millions of men and women as homogeneous: and thus treats black people as particularized expressions of a racial essence—as tokens of a human type—in precisely the way invented by nineteenth century extrinsic racism" (emphasis added).[76] In any case, every individual will belong to many groups and her perspectives on life will be shaped by all of them. We never say all that is important, or even that which is most important, about a person when we classify her racially or ethnically. A self-image that is limited to race is an impoverished one.[77]

Toward an active self-image

While an individual's perspective, to the extent that it is a black one, will be shaped by aspects of black experience, it is important to insure that it is not only our experiences as victims that matter.[78] One is struck on reading Flack and Pellegrino, Sanders, Murray, and others by how overwhelmingly negative are the experiences they cite as shaping our perspective: slavery and discrimination, our experience as an oppressed people, dehumanization, and poverty. Only a fool would deny the weight of these experiences. But we must recognize that a perspective shaped exclusively by suffering is bound to be severely distorted. A conscious effort, then, must be made to emphasize more positive elements of our experience as African-Americans.[79] Even then it will not be enough to stress the good things that have happened to us; we must also view ourselves as agents in the world, as beings with power (severely limited but real power), as Kant said, to make the world conform to our vision.[80]

Establishing community limits

If we are correct in following the communitarians who understand a real community to be a group united in pursuit of a shared vision of life, then we must abandon the romantic idea that everyone within a certain geographic area or with a certain skin color is a member of an African-American community. The dope-peddler, the pimp, the gang member, the mugger, or at least the adults among them, are not *in* the community but against it. Those not-yet adult members of this fringe may be community members insofar as someone pledges allegiance to its goals on their behalf, I suppose, rather in the way some religious traditions understand infant baptism. But the adults are out. This is not to repeat the mistake of those who insist some African-Americans are not really black, or to retrieve the demand I earlier rejected for a uniform racial "party line." My point is simply that not every African-American is really a member of some African-American community.[81] (In the same way, we recognize that not everyone who is by descent a member of a certain family is contributing to the family's joint project of helping one another to attain better lives; some are doing the opposite.) Clarity is not advanced by blinding ourselves to these facts. While there can be great differences within a community about the means to be used in pursuit of the shared vision as well as differences of taste and style, there are limits.[82]

Recognizing cultural limits

There is a tendency at present to limit the notion of "culture" to the recent meaning used and popularized by social scientists: a group's "way of life" together.[83] Perhaps that notion does have some usefulness, although it is exceedingly vague. It is, however, a mistake to use this term exclusively in a sense that divorces it from its ancient meaning and etymology, which connect it to "agriculture," "soil-cultivation," and even "cell culture" (and ultimately to being a "cultivated" or "cultured" person). When we think of African-American culture in its most proper and central sense, we should think of what *nurtures* and *develops* us as people (and therein as *a* people), of what improves us and helps us mature, to develop.[84] Across groups and across individuals, there will, of course, be different beliefs about the details of culture, and sometimes it may be difficult to know which ideas are correct. Nonetheless, there is no reason to accept as "culture" in the deeper sense that which merely debases, panders to, or destroys us.[85]

When we think about "culture" in this richer way, we should find ourselves less likely to follow Professor Gates who seemingly wants to make a case that even the vilest lyrics written and performed by the singing group Two Live Crew are part of African-American culture because they are the modern representative of a "street tradition."[86] Whereas their lyrics may place them in an African-American "way of life" in some broad sense, talk of "culture" should help us draw a crucial distinction between ways of living, of being vital and contributing to growth, on the one hand, and ways of dying, of degenerating and of sinking into corruption, on the other.

Similarly, we need to avoid a related error bequeathed from shallow social science, especially one infected with myths of a logical "gap" between facts and values and the possibility of a "value free" science of human experience. That error is the tendency to identify a culture with what people actually do, to the neglect of the ideals and goals they espouse. It is, of course, tempting to dismiss the latter as mere dishonesty and hypocrisy. A culture, however, must be the culture of some community and, as we observed above, communities exist only when people are tied one to another in common pursuits and a shared vision of what they wish to become. Thus, we may miss precisely what unites a group, what makes its individuals into one people, when we disregard the aspirations, ambitions, and objectives that they hold both for themselves as individuals and for their common life.

When our ethical standpoint is shaped by some determinate vision of that richer and more serious notion of culture, then our options might look very different to us. We might, for example, begin to see that among the features of African-American culture most worth saving are such elements as the tradition of strong females, the special values accorded children, the sort of religious life that extends beyond Sunday observances, strong cross-generational ties, and the misgivings about wealth and power borne of having been victims of their abuse. Some of these are survivals of our African past; others arose in response to the exigencies of slavery and its aftermath; all will need to be adapted to our changing circumstances. Unfortunately, these are among the aspects of African-American life most often neglected and even scorned by black intellectuals.

POSTRADICAL AFRICAN-AMERICAN CONSCIOUSNESS

A final point. If the notions of black identity and consciousness are still to be useful, the time is long since past to free them from the 1960s. DuBois wrote of the complex duality built into our status as African-Americans.[87] Too often, one finds black writers seeming to reduce this complexity to a pair of easy equations, exalting in and encouraging what is African in us, while condemning the American as bad and something to be expunged.[88] It is not, I submit, as simple as that.

It is said that we are Africans in diaspora. But this is, at best, misleading. We are people of African descent, which is something very different. Even Africans are not merely Africans. As the African-born philosopher Appiah reminds us, "the peoples of Africa have a good deal less culturally in common than is usually assumed."[89] The violence between Buthelezi's followers and Mandela's may be grim testimony to his point.

It is said that we and all nonwhite peoples make up the Third World. But if there is such a world, it is not a united one. Black people boycott Korean grocers in Brooklyn; Japanese officials make racist remarks. Africans oppress Africans and Arabs, Arabs.

At a time when Castro and Deng stand as holdout dictators while the tides of liberation sweep the world, it should be clear that the black radicals who imagined, and sometimes still imagine, themselves kindred revolutionaries of Che and Mao are not only dreamers, but that their dream is a nightmare. At a time when the economic question is more the transition from communism to capitalism than the other way around, and when America and its symbols stand as signs of liberation from the Berlin Wall to Lithuania, from Moscow to Beijing, reflexive anti-Americanism is, to use a word over-used (and misused) in the 1960s, irrelevant.[90] Charles Johnson anticipates the day when we will read a work of fiction by Americans "who happen to be black [and who] feel at ease both in their ethnicity and in their Yankeeness. . . ."[91] That day is not yet here, and we are not yet ready for it, but working toward such a goal can be part of a new and postradical black self-understanding.[92]

Preston Williams once wrote of black people proceeding through stages from (1) victimization, through (2) the sporadic "integration" among reluctant white people of a few extraordinary black individuals as exceptions to the exclusionist rule, to (3) the time of black awareness.[93] The time may be ripe for conceptualizing a fourth stage, one in which we operate comfortably within this society, each of us with his or her individual problems, but all of us accepted as, and pleased to be, members in good standing. Then we will have realized DuBois's vision of a time when the African-American's "double self" will have merged "into a better and truer self."

NOTES

1. This paper was prepared for presentation to an interdisciplinary symposium, "African-American Perspectives on Biomedical Ethics" at Georgetown University, December 10-12, 1990. Doctors Pellegrino and Flack showed great confidence in me in inviting me to speak on these topics at the intersection of African-American Studies and medical ethics, two areas in which I have more interest than expertise and on which I had not previously

tried to articulate my thoughts. Professors William Banner and Tom Beauchamp helped me by providing thoughtful commentaries at the conference session as did the questions and comments from the conference participants. Dennis McManus assisted me in preparing this manuscript for publication. To all of them I am grateful.

All quotations in this paragraph are from William Banner, "Is there an African-American Perspective on Biomedical Ethics?" presented at the Georgetown Conference and included in this volume.

2. The extramental, so conceived, approximates (closely enough, I hope, for our purposes) some standard accounts of what British and American philosophers have lately called "realism." (See the introduction and essays collected in Geoffrey Sayre-McCord, ed. *Moral Realism* [Ithaca, New York: Cornell University Press, 1988]).

Cultural relativism as I define it here is to be distinguished from moral skepticism, the thesis that no real knowledge of right and wrong or good and evil is attainable.

3. The idea and terminology for the first two theses I borrow from John Ladd's introduction to *Ethical Relativism* (ed. John Ladd [Belmont, California: Wadsworth Publishing Co., 1973], 1-11). The idea, and awkward terminology, for the third is my own. I add this thesis to reserve the term "cultural relativist" for those who think that ultimately there is no legitimate and objective basis on which to rank and choose among cultures, and to distinguish such thinkers from those I call "communitarians" who, while strongly linking morality to tradition, insist upon the ability for such rational appraisal and choice. My terminology is probably somewhat idiosyncratic, but not without some rationale.

4. See, e.g., Bernard Williams, *Ethics and the Limits of Philosophy* (Cambridge, Massachusetts: Harvard University Press, 1985); Stuart Hampshire, "Morality and Convention," in *Morality and Conflict* (Cambridge, Massachusetts: Harvard University Press, 1983), 126-139.

5. Many social scientists seem to subscribe to this combination of relativism and functionalism. Alain Locke, e.g., writes approvingly of Pareto's "historical and functional relativism of cultural values," and concludes the most important of his philosophical essays, "Values and Imperatives," by invoking "a new center for the thought and insight of our present generation . . . a philosophy and a psychology, and perhaps too, a sociology, pivoted around functionalistic relativism" (Alain Locke, "Values and Imperatives," in *Philosophy Born of Struggle*, ed. Leonard Harris [Dubuque, Iowa: Kendall-Hunt, 1983], 32, 34).

6. The first assessment of Locke is from Leonard Harris's introduction to *Philosophy Born of Struggle*, xiii. The self-assessment is from Locke's autobiographical note accompanying his "Values and Imperatives," p. 35. My exposition relates entirely to Locke's views as presented in this essay, his most significant piece of academic philosophical writing. Professor Leonard Harris has suggested to me that in other works Locke's position appears more subtle and nuanced than the cultural relativism of "Values and Imperatives."

7.   Johnny Washington, "Alain L. Locke's 'Values and Imperatives': An Interpretation" in *Philosophy Born of Struggle*, 155.

8.   Alain Locke, "Values and Imperatives," in *Philosophy Born of Struggle*, 32.

9.   Ibid., 31.

10.   Ibid., 31.

11.   Ibid., 27-30. It is both surprising and unfortunate that Locke is silent on the corresponding feud in the last of his four fields of value—the moral. According to him, the introverted type of emotional response in this field constitutes the realm of ethical ideals, is expressed in terms of the good and the bad, and concerns the struggle between conscience and temptation; the extroverted type constitutes the realm of interpersonal morality, is expressed in terms of the right and the wrong, and concerns the struggle between duty and crime.

This view prefigures Peter Strawson's influential distinction between the social realm of morality and the private realm of personal ethical ideals in his "Social Morality and Individual Ideal," in *The Definition of Morality*, ed. Gerald Wallace and A. D. M. Walker (London: Methuen, 1970), 98-119. That distinction, in various forms, is the heart of the new neutralist political morality some American and British philosophers espouse, according to which the liberal state properly concerns itself with moral questions of right and wrong in persons' dealings with one another (especially in their collective distribution of benefits and burdens), but is expected to maintain strict neutrality toward the various personal ethical ideals of the different individuals within a modern pluralistic society.

12.   Locke, "Values and Imperatives," 29.

13.   Ibid., 32.

14.   Here again Locke seems to have anticipated a topic that has recently drawn considerable attention. Some philosophers have complained about the alleged tendency of religious and of moral values to claim a rank for themselves that makes it seem base to take time away from them for the pursuit of values in other fields. See Bernard Williams, *Ethics and the Limits*; and Michael A. Slote, *Goods and Virtues* (Oxford: Clarendon Press, 1983).

15.   For a startlingly negative re-appraisal of the Negritude movement, see Charles Johnson, *Being and Race: Black Writing since 1917* (Bioomington, Indiana: Indiana University Press, 1988), 18-23. Compare Alain Locke's own essay, "The New Negro," in *Philosophy Born of Struggle*, 242-251.

16.   Locke, "Values and Imperatives," 32.

17.   I have presented these arguments with a little more detail in my "Relativism and Moral Divergence." The general anti-relativist strategy resembles that of Donald Davidson's in "On the Very Idea of a Conceptual Scheme," *Relativism: Cognitive and Moral*, ed. Jack W. Meiland and Michael Krausz (Notre Dame: University of Notre Dame Press, 1982).

For some early and influential criticisms of formal criteria of morality, see Philippa Foot's "Moral Beliefs" and "Moral Arguments" in her *Virtues and Vices* (Berkeley: University of California Press, 1978).

18. This undermines at least some versions of the position called "cultural equity," which holds that all cultures are of equal value. It is hard to know how to assign a single value to a whole culture and, once such assignments are made, it is incredible to suppose that, for any two cultures, C1 and C2, the value of C1 will be exactly equal to that of C2. Of course, in general, it will be difficult to judge the value of a culture as a whole. Often, however, it is not difficult to judge how well a culture is doing in this or that respect, e.g., in providing for the health or liberty of the people living in it. And surely a culture that does a bad enough job in all the pertinent areas can properly be said to be worse on the whole than one that better succeeds in all of them. Perhaps what the proponents of cultural equity mean to say is that all cultures are equally valueless in the sense that there are no true judgments of the comparative value of two cultures. Many philosophers, influenced by logical positivism, used to think that value judgments lacked truth because they had a special kind of meaning that made them more like imperatives or ejaculations than like statements of fact. This claim, however, makes it extremely difficult to explain the logical behavior of value judgments and the thesis of cultural equity is indeed insecure if its fate depends on such discredited theories of language.

Some maintain that African-American culture is not merely equal but superior to its chief domestic rival. Sanders maintains that the African-American ethos is "humanistic in ways that the European-American ethos is not" (see her "Problems and Limitations of an African-American Perspective in Biomedical Ethics, A theological View," in this volume). And according to unsympathetic press reports, Leonard Jeffries holds Nazism to be the ultimate culmination of the white value system, which supposedly derives from deformation of white genes during the Ice Ages, while blacks hold "the value system of the sun" (see Dinesh D'Souza, "Illiberal Education," *The Atlantic*, 267 (March, 1991): 54).

Of course, people shouldn't make remarks of this nature unless they have the best of evidence, and even then they shouldn't make them without some qualification to disavow any suggestion that African-Americans are themselves more human than European-Americans. Still, it is possible and even likely that some cultures will, in some of their aspects, surpass others, and it is surely romantic to imagine that all these factors will even out so as to leave every culture on the whole exactly equal to every other one. The art journalist Peggy Cooper Cafritz claims to hold some version of this thesis of cultural equity, but I do not know whether her version runs afoul of the arguments I adduced here.

19. See note 4.

20. An important recent collection of essays representing the state of the current discussion on cultural relativism is Michael Krausz, ed., *Relativism: Interpretation and Confrontation* (Notre Dame: University of Notre Dame Press, 1989). In his introduction (p. 2), Krausz notes, in addition to the kind of relativism we have discussed, the possibility of a "nonframework" relativism, which holds that "more than one uniquely correct interpretation"

may apply to a given domain of objects (or of discourse), "on account of a multiplicity of standards." I won't pursue that sort of relativism here, since it need have no important connection to matters of culture and ethnicity; however, we should note the difficulty of making intelligible the claim that there can be *more than one* interpretation that is *uniquely* correct.

21.   Alain Locke's view that his relativistic "pluralism" somehow supports a principle of tolerance is disturbingly close to the position Bernard Williams rightly castigates as "vulgar relativism" in his *Morality: An Introduction to Ethics* (New York: Harper & Row, 1972), 20.

22.   Strictly speaking, a perspective is the view one gets, how things look to one, from a standpoint. To introduce a little linguistic variation, I shall cheat a bit, sometimes using the terms "point of view," "vantage point," and "standpoint" to mean the same thing.

23.   The procedure outlined is a generally Kantian picture. For a discussion that articulates the limits of this process of objectification, imaginatively extends this picture of the construction of the objective order to cover a variety of philosophical issues, and stresses the constant danger that such a process will lead us to undervalue the subjective order, see Thomas Nagel, *The View from Nowhere* (New York: Oxford University Press, 1986).

24.   Compare the assumption implicit in this quotation from a report on revising New York State school curricula to make them multicultural. "The subject matter should be treated as socially constructed and therefore tentative—as is all knowledge" (Quoted in an editorial, "Mr. Sobol's Planet," *The New Republic* [July, 15 and 22, 1991]: 5-6). Someone's knowing certain facts, e.g., about astronomy or history, will result from her biochemistry as well as from her physical and cultural environment, but it does not follow that the scientific or historical facts she knows are at all determined by her culture.

The tendency to make an unwarranted leap from a recognition of the fact that human cognition is shaped by culture and history, to the fanciful claim that reality itself is a human construct is an old one that has exerted undue influence in Western philosophy, since at least the time of Leibniz and Berkeley. Ontology, however, is not, and cannot be read as epistemology, still less as cognitive psychology or the sociology of belief. It appears that quite a few proponents of multiculturalism merely give familiar brands of relativism a thoroughly Western pedigree, when they could have helped us transcend this contingent and parochial academic fashion. The same holds for the allied attempt to see every culture through the prism of "race, class, and gender," a clump of preoccupations that have come to the fore in the West under the influence of a specific group of Western intellectual and social movements. If multiculturalism contains the truth that will set us free, it would do well to break these bonds.

25.   Future work on ethnic perspectives in ethics should be informed by parallel work on gender perspectives. Female natural scientists do not study a different physical world from the one males study, but it is not at all difficult to suppose that their different experiences (to say nothing of biochemical differences) might attract women in disproportionate numbers to certain

problems, methodologies, types of theory. This could even lead to different scientific views predominating within each gender group. What it couldn't lead to is two opposed scientific claims both being true, and what it shouldn't distract us from is the fact that ultimately the natural scientist, whether female or male, seeks to find out about our single shared physical universe. In science and in ethics, we seek the truth. For an overview of writings on women in the sciences and in the philosophy of science, see Clifford Geertz, "A Lab of One's Own," *New York Review of Books* 37 (November 8, 1990): 19-23; and Margarita Levin, "Feminists and Science," *American Scholar* (Winter, 1988): 100-106.

26. Cheryl Sanders, "Problems and Limitations," in this volume.

27. I do not mean to imply that either race or ethnicity is properly a category of natural science. I doubt that either is. Janet Helms is aware of the problem posed by the indeterminate boundaries of race classifications, but nonetheless borrows a biological definition of race from the 1940s as "a sub-group of peoples possessing a definite combination of physical characters, of genetic origin, the combination of which to varying degrees distinguishes the sub-group from other sub-groups of mankind." Faced with this sort of thinking, one wants to ask what biological features are necessary, in what degrees, and in which acceptable combinations for one to be, for example, a member of the black race. Would facial hair curled to tightness M1, say, suffice to offset a melanin content as low as M2? (Janet Helms, *Black and White Racial Identity: Theory, Research, and Practice* [New York: Greenwood Press, 1990], 3).

On race as unscientific, see Kwame Anthony Appiah, "The Uncompleted Argument: DuBois and the Illusion of Race," *"Race," Writing, and Difference*, ed. Henry Louis Gates (Chicago: University of Chicago Press, 1986), 21-37.

Items from the history of racial classification in the natural and social sciences are briefly sketched in Raymond Williams, *Keywords* (New York: Oxford, 1983 revised ed.), *s.vv.* "Ethnic" and "Racial." See also Lucius Outlaw, "Toward a Critical Theory of 'Race,'" and H. L. Gates, "Critical Remarks," in *Anatomy of Racism*, ed. David T. Goldberg (Minneapolis: University of Minnesota Press, 1990), 58-82 and 319-329, respectively.

My point is that the best unscientific criteria we have for applying these unscientific terms are not psychological ones but physical and historical ones. Surprisingly, several writers appear to jump from this claim that race is not a natural-scientific classification to the stronger thesis that race is not real, making a point, for example, scrupulously to place the term between quotation marks. This inference and the orthographic practice associated with it seem to be unwarranted. After all, one would be hard-pressed to defend the claim that several concepts thought important in ethics, such as those of person, intention, value, desire, welfare, are scientific. For a related discussion, see David Wiggins, "Truth, Invention, and the Meaning of Life," in his *Needs, Values, and Truth* (Oxford: Basil Blackwell, 1987).

28. Frantz Fanon, "The Fact of Blackness," in *Anatomy of Racism*, 121. For another existentialist-informed criticism of attempts to constrain us within a supposed black essence, see Charles Johnson, *Being and Race*.

29.   It sometimes seems that certain thinkers want to take their politics from optics: the more a person and her statements indicate reflection (e.g., by showing independence of thought, interest in topics or goals other than those of advancement, sensitivity to issues outside a prescribed political compass), the less black they are. (For complaints comparable to mine, see Shelby Steele, *The Content of Our Character* [New York: St. Martin's Press, 1990]; Stanley Crouch, *Notes of a Hanging Judge* [New York: Oxford University Press, 1990]; Charles Johnson, *Being and Race*.) One wonders: do we need a new term for the practice these writers condemn? Or should we perhaps renovate the old term "denigrate," teasing out of its prefix, root, and suffix the new meaning "to un-blacken"?

If I understand it aright, part of the point of an autobiographical text that Professor Adrian Piper incorporated into one of her art works is that one way in which white racism can permeate the mind of its victims is in forcing a person of mixed ancestry to think it a matter of great moment that she decide, once and for all, whether she is white *or* black. Reportedly, Nazis used elaborate genealogical research to determine a person's race, while South Africa under apartheid preferred investigations of her fingernails, hair, and cheekbone structure. Given the arbitrariness of racial classification and the fuzzy boundaries of race concepts, a sensible answer to the question "Are you black or white?" might be "Some of each." Or, lest that bring social scientists on the run with "instruments" to measure one's degree of "negrescence," it might be better to ask in response, "What hangs on it?" (Professor Piper's piece, "Political Self-Portrait #3" (1980) appeared in an exhibition *Adrian Piper: Reflections 1967-1987* at the Washington Project for the Arts, 1991.)

Of course, in a more vicious phase of racism, the racists might arrogate this power of classification to themselves. A classic novel from James Weldon Johnson offers a psychological study of the effect of one attempt, through deceit, to escape a socially-imposed racial classification. At its close, the "ex-colored man," who "passes" for white, says of the "small but gallant band of colored men who are publicly fighting the cause of their race" that "Beside them I feel small and selfish. I am an ordinarily successful white man who has made a little money. They are men who are making history and a race. I, too, might have taken part in a work so glorious. . . . I cannot repress the thought that, after all, I have chosen the lesser part, that I have sold my birthright for a mess of pottage" (See James Weldon Johnson, *The Autobiography of an Ex-Colored Man* reprinted in *Three Negro Classics* [New York: Avon Books, 1965], especially 510-511).

A related piece by Professor Piper, "Political Self-Portrait #2" (1979), records the even more painful pressure toward racial identification and self-definition that other African-Americans exerted as she was growing up, mocking her as "Paleface" and chastising her for socializing with white people and "acting too white." In a similar vein, in Spike Lee's 1991 film *Jungle Fever*, the (black) character Flipper derides children of mixed racial ancestry as themselves "mixed up . . . mixed nuts." Flipper's (white) mistress correctly dismisses as "racist" these sentiments, ugly in themselves and cruel in the context.

Perhaps worst of all, efforts to measure how black a person and his or her ideas are sometimes consist in taking as normative types of behavior, attitudes, and political positions that perpetuate forms of degradation that originated in oppression, that are self-destructive, and that trade on increasingly *passé* paradigms of inter-group relations. Even Janet Helms, a psychologist who allows that a person at the "most developed" stage of "Black racial identity" will achieve the sort of "racial transcendence" that facilitates, in her jargon, a "reference group orientation" that is "bicultural [and] pluralistic," cautiously says only that such a person can "reestablish relationships with *individual* White associates who *merit*" them (Janet Helms, *Black and White Racial Identity*, 30, 29; emphases added). This plainly presupposes that black people will normally confront white ones, not only as different, but as antagonists.

30.   A. MacIntyre is the leading figure in this movement, but my general characterization of this position is not meant faithfully to represent the views of any particular communitarian thinker. Nevertheless, see Alasdair MacIntyre, *After Virtue* (Notre Dame: University of Notre Dame Press, 1981), and *Whose Justice? Which Rationality?* (Notre Dame: University of Notre Dame Press, 1988).

MacIntyre himself has recently denied that he is a communitarian but his reasons, namely, that "the political, economic, and moral structures of advanced modernity . . . exclude the possibility of realizing any of the worthwhile types of political community . . . [and because] attempts to remake modern societies in systematically communitarian ways will always be either ineffective or disastrous," do not preclude his being a communitarian as I am using the term. They imply merely that he will be unhappy with modern society and pessimistic about improving it. (See Alasdair MacIntyre, "I'm Not a Communitarian, But . . ." *Responsive Community* 1 [Summer, 1991]: 91-92. I am grateful to Terry Pinkard for this reference.)

31.   I follow some leading communitarians in expressing their thought in terms of diverse "traditions" rather than in terms of "codes," because some of them stress that a community's moral life is often best understood as a matter of conformity to established models rather than following some specified set of regulations. These models or ideals may focus not on behavior so much as on meaning: what sort of person to be, how to live, what goals to adopt, which interests, tastes, and feelings to cultivate and which to curb. Thus MacIntyre, and other communitarians of this tendency, contribute to the resurgence of philosophical interest in the virtues.

32.   Charles Olson, "These Days," in C. Olson, *Collected Poems* (Berkeley: University of California Press, 1987).

33.   Alasdair MacIntyre, *After Virtue*, especially chaps. 2, 3.

34.   "There is no such thing as *man* in the world. In the course of my life I have seen Frenchmen, Italians, Russians, etc.; I know too, thanks to Montesquieu, that one can be a Persian. But as for Man, I declare I have never

met him in my life; if he exists, he is unknown to me" (Joseph de Maistre, *Considerations sur la France* [1875]. Translated by and quoted in Isaiah Berlin, "Joseph de Maistre and the Origins of Fascism, I." *New York Review of Books* 37, Nr. 14 [September 27, 1990]: 59). Berlin has recently argued that de Maistre, for all his reactionary prose, is in fact a herald of what some might call *postmodernist* thinking, and a writer unjustly neglected at a time when philosophical attacks on rationalist and humanist thought again have currency (see Isaiah Berlin, "Joseph de Maistre and the Origins of Fascism, II, III," *New York Review of Books*, 37, No. 15 [October 11, 1990], 54-58, and 37, No. 16 [October 25, 1990], 61-65).

35.   For a helpful summary of two influential communitarian works, a discussion that focuses precisely on this process of critical renewal of a culture, see two reviews by Martha Nussbaum, "Recoiling from Reason," *New York Review of Books* (December 7, 1989), 36-41; and "Review of Charles Taylor's 'Sources of the Self,'" *New Republic*.

36.   Indeed, communitarianism as I use the term could be considered a particularly weak form of relativism though, for purposes of exposition, it best serves as an alternative to, rather than a version of, cultural relativism.

37.   Cheryl Sanders, "Problems and Limitations," in this volume.

38.   It should go without saying that the more important questions about a belief are whether it is true and whether it is epistemically reasonable, and the more important question about a desire or an emotive response is whether it is decent morally.

39.   Contrast the view of Professor Ronald Walters who, in the course of criticizing the conservative political views of Judge Clarence Thomas and opposing his nomination to the United States Supreme Court, remarks: "His views are unrepresentative [of those of most black people in the United States]. In this sense, he will be found not to be the 'black' nominee to the court, because *'blackness' ultimately means more than color, it also means a set of values* from which Thomas is estranged" ("Thomas: Estranged from his 'Blackness,'" *Washington Post*, July 15, 1991, A11, emphasis added). My contention is that "blackness" cannot mean any specific set of values, though we may reasonably say that a certain individual's ethical commitments are more or less greatly influenced by experiences she or he has had precisely because she or he is an African-American. This is a matter of the history of the individual's coming to have ethical commitments, not of which commitments she has (*pace* Walters), or the type of rational justification available to her.

40.   Dinesh D'Souza, *Illiberal Education*, 187, 206. The scholar D'Souza here criticizes is Thomas Kochman, who according to D'Souza (p. 296), says that black people (1) "do not believe that emotions interfere with their capacity to reason," (2) treat debate opponents "as antagonists, givers and receivers of abuse," (3) see political motives behind "the requirement to behave, calmly and rationally, when negotiating," (4) are wont to "approach black women in a manner that openly expresses sexual interest." These quotations are taken out of context, but even a cursory examination of Kochman's book indicates that he does sometimes deal in stereotypes; e.g.,

"Within black culture, the rules of rapping maintain that a woman can be approached and hit on at any time and place" (T. Kochman, *Black and White: Styles in Conflict* [Chicago: University of Chicago Press, 1981], 87). Indeed, even Kochman's explanation that, for him, the term "black" "represents the ethnic patterns and perspectives of black 'community' people, called elsewhere *ghetto blacks, inner-city blacks*, or *Afro-Americans*" (p. 14), serves to confirm the charge that his conception of black people is stereotyped, thus substantiating Shelby Steele's complaint that, to some, only poor black people are really black.

41.   Helms, *Black and White Racial Identity*, 17.

42.   Ibid., appendices 2 and 3.

43.   Ibid., 5, 85. Why it should be thought psychologically advanced to try to conform one's "feelings, thoughts, and behavior" to those of other members of a racial group is not addressed. Any epistemological or ethical theory that held one's beliefs or conduct to be epistemically or morally justified by such conformity would plainly be bankrupt.

44.   Ibid., 86.

45.   For a different developmental approach to the question of culturally-informed ethical perspectives, one developed in critical reaction to the work of Lawrence Kohlberg, see Anthony Cortese, *Ethnic Ethics* (Albany: State University of New York Press, 1990), chapters 2, 5.

46.   Annette Dula, "Yes, there are African-American Perspectives on Bioethics," in this volume. My thinking on these topics, especially in this section of the text, has been greatly influenced by this paper.

47.   Harley Flack and Edmund Pellegrino, "New Data Suggests African-Americans Have Own Perspective On Biomedical Ethics," *Kennedy Institute Newsletter*, vol. 3, No. 2 (April, 1989): 2.

48.   That, perhaps, is a part of what Dula means when she says that African-American perspectives will be shaped not only by our experience of health care but also by our "distinctive world view" and our "history of unequal power relations—a history of oppression, domination and subordination, of ridicule" ("Yes, There are," in this volume).

49.   Permit me one observation. One figure in the health care industry about, and from, whom we hear very little in discussions of bioethics is the service worker. If, as I have suggested, one of the benefits of identifying and understanding overlooked perspectives on a set of topics is to correct for the distortion caused by always viewing those topics from the same point of view, then one of the ways in which heeding African-American perspectives may be most useful to the field of bioethics may be precisely in allowing the voices of the service worker, the orderly, the nurse's aide, the driver, and janitor, to be heard. African-Americans are likely to be disproportionately represented among such nonprofessional laborers in the health care industry. Plainly, these workers are affected by, and need to be heard on, decisions about hospital financing. It may also be that listening to the one whose job it is (for example) to discard aborted fetuses, will help us gain insight into what we are doing in some medical procedures.

A further, more personal, note. Before I ever gave a thought to medicine or medical ethics, I encountered the health care distribution system via the many members of my family who worked at major urban hospitals in meal preparation, operating elevators, as messenger, and as supply-room laborer. They were members of a hospital employees' union, both my parents serving as delegates in Local 1199. The hospital in which they worked eventually bought the tenement in which we lived, raised the rents, then razed the building in which I was reared, along with three-quarters of the other structures on the block, to provide parking space. This, doubtless, was supposed to enable the institution to better serve the community it had thereby destroyed. Thus, in my youth, I experienced the medical center as an unfair employer, oppressive institutional neighbor, absentee landlord, and, eventually, agent of eviction. I don't deny that this experience has "colored" my view of such institutions. I suggest, however, that adopting the perspectives of the service employee, the neighborhood resident, and the tenant, can alert us to a new array of ethical questions involving health care institutions— questions usually ignored.

50.   Cheryl Sanders, "Problems and Limitations," in this volume. See also Robert Murray, "Minority Perspectives on Biomedical Ethics," unpublished paper presented at a Fidia Foundation Symposium: "Transcultural Dimensions of Medical Ethics," Washington, D.C. (April 26-27, 1990), 5-10.

51.   It seems to me that philosophical work should have logical, methodological, and hierarchical priority over the sociological, but that may be merely professional bias.

52.   For a summary of contemporary utilitarianism, see the editors' introduction in *Utilitarianism and Beyond*, ed. Amartya Sen and Bernard Williams (Cambridge: Cambridge University Press, 1982). "Direct utilitarianism" requires agents to perform those actions which themselves have the best results; "indirect utilitarianism" requires them to perform those actions which are somehow tied to something else (rules, principles, traits of character) general observance or possession of which would have the best results.

One classic statement of the view is John Stuart Mill, *Utilitarianism*. Early utilitarianism is associated with the principle that one ought to perform the action that will bring about the greatest good to the greatest number of persons. More recent writers have found this principle viciously ambiguous and tend to prefer a form of the principle that omits the final prepositional phrase. (For a treatment of some worries about ambiguity, see Nicholas Rescher, *Distributive Justice*, [Indianapolis: Bobbs-Merrill, 1966]).

It is worth noting, that these latter-day utilitarians are not logically committed to majoritarianism. If, for example, no action will produce more than N units of good, but action X will share this good with a number of people while action Y will give it all to me, then nothing in the principle that the agent maximize the total good produced requires her to choose X over Y. Nonetheless, most philosophers today would favor a moral theory that supplemented the principle requiring agents to maximize good with an additional principle requiring them to favor the larger number of beneficiaries, at least in cases of ties.

53.   Robert M. Veatch, "Allocating Organs by Utilitarianism Is Seen as Favoring Whites Over Blacks," *Kennedy Institute of Ethics Newsletter*, 3 (July, 1989): 1, 3.

54.   Ibid., 3.

55.   *Malcolm X Speaks*, (New York: Grove Press, 1966), 133, 136. Four months prior to this December 1964 address, Barry Goldwater accepted the Republican presidential nomination in a speech famous for the line, "Moderation in the pursuit of justice is no virtue. Extremism in the defense of liberty is no vice."

56.   See C. M. Francis, "Conflicts and Confluences: Ancient and Modern Medical Ethics in India," Fidia Foundation Conference: "Transcultural Dimensions of Medical Ethics," Washington, D.C. (April 26-27, 1990), 5.

57.   That this sort of initiative is often urged by some of today's so-called "ethicists" may indicate that behind the placid mask of Apollo, which these self-proclaimed proponents of reason prefer to sport, there gape the jaws of Moloch.

58.   Murray, "Minority Perspectives," 6.

59.   I do not mean to deny that affirmative action to increase the representation of African-Americans among health care professionals is needed. That, of course, raises the vexed questions of preferential treatment in hiring and in professional school admissions, which has recently come under criticism from some black intellectuals, not only such conservatives as Professor Thomas Sowell, but also Professors Shelby Steele and William Julius Wilson, among others. I cannot discuss these matters in any detail here. Permit me, however, a few observations.

First, even when one ultimate goal of a program of preferential treatment is simply to help its immediate beneficiaries, it is not aimed at punishing wrongdoers. Thus, frequently-heard complaints that white applicants who lose positions to black ones are themselves innocent of racist practice and attitudes, even when true, miss the point. William Raspberry, himself an opponent of many forms of affirmative action, has offered a useful analogy with veterans' benefits that were encouraged and widely accepted in the United States after World War II (William Raspberry, discussion on *Mac-Neil/Lehrer Report*, June 14, 1991). There were, of course, female and handicapped applicants who were deprived of benefits because of these preference programs, even though they were "innocent" in that it was no fault of their own that they had failed to serve in the military. That does nothing, however, to show that the programs were unjust. The one who lost out never had a *right* to be hired or admitted; employers and schools could properly use their hiring and admissions policies to advance any number of legitimate and relevant objectives. Indeed, without these programs the female or handicapped applicant might have enjoyed an unearned advantage over veterans who missed out on training while serving. These programs were a morally licit way for society to express its appreciation for the sacrifices the veterans had made on its behalf. As a society may be indebted to members of group X for the good they have done and for the sacrifices they have suffered, so may a society owe something to members of group Y for the wrong it has done them or for the ills they suffer because of wrongs it has done to others. Preferential treatment should not be seen solely or even primarily as reparations, but I do think that reparations are part of the rationale for such programs. And even though the white applicant who loses a position may be "innocent," it is difficult to see how he or she is being treated unjustly. As in the veterans' parallel case, without the program of preferential treatment, the white applicant would enjoy an unearned edge over the person whom the effects of slavery, discrimination and racism, have placed at a disadvantage in the applicant pool.

Second, although being hired or admitted can be an advantage to the one who gets it, what we have just said shows that it is a mistake to think of positions in schools and workplaces as prizes to be awarded to deserving winners. As the term's etymology indicates (*de servir* "from serving"), desert is always a backward-looking matter, a matter of what one has done or been. Admission and hiring, on the other hand, are incentives and opportunities that are distributed with an eye to the future. While it is patently absurd to dismiss the whole idea of qualifications and merit, there is reason to protest the sharp distinction commonly assumed between considerations of diversification and considerations of merit. An applicant is qualified or merits selection insofar as hiring or admitting her advances the goals we are trying to promote in filling the slot. It may well be an important contribution to an individual's learning or working experience that she be exposed to, and come to appreciate, differing points of view; and one important way to insure this experience is to build an ethnically diverse educational and working environment. The same is obviously true of health care professionals, who will often be working with and treating people of diverse backgrounds. The fact that a given applicant for a position in a medical or nursing school or care-facility—Applicant #1, for example—will help contribute to such an ambience is itself, therefore, a consideration in favor of hiring her; it makes her a better choice, other things being equal. Thus, we should not rush to infer that because another candidate, Applicant #2, has better test scores, Applicant #2 is eo ipso better qualified than, and merits selection over, Applicant #1.

By the way, it is merely a non sequitur to think, as D'Souza seems to do, that one who believes that increasing ethnic diversity is likely to increase diversity of outlooks must suppose that all members of a given group think alike (Dinesh D'Souza, *Illiberal Education*, 53). The second chapter of D'Souza's book helpfully reports some conversations about the virtues and vices of preferential university admissions. For application of a general philosophical account of desert to discussions of affirmative action, see J. L. A. Garcia, "A Problem about the Basis of Desert," *Journal of Social Philosophy* 19 (1988): 11-19.

60. "Boarder babies [are] children abandoned by crack-addicted mothers and left for hospitals to rear or place in foster homes." See Michele

Norris's reports on children who themselves or whose parents are addicted to "crack" cocaine, "Suffering the Sins of the Mother," *Washington Post*, June 30, 1991, 1, 16; "Love Spoken Here," and "Brief High Creates a Lifetime of Loss," Ibid., 17. Norris reports that 30 percent of the 1400 babies born at Howard University Hospital in 1990 had been exposed to drugs *in utero*.

61.   Bowman cites statistics from the Department of Health and Human Services, according to which, as he interprets them, "in the white population, the number of abortions per 100 live births was 17.5 percent in 1973 and 31.2 percent in 1981. Blacks constituted the vast majority of the 'all others' group. In this group the abortions per 100 live births in 1973 were 28.9 percent and, in 1981, 54.4 percent" (James E. Bowman, "The Plight of Poor African-Americans: Public Policy on Sickle Hemoglobin and AIDS," in this volume, p. 00). Bowman's statistics are from "Health in the United States, 1984," DHHS Publication number (PHS) 85-1232. It should be noted that most estimates put the ratio of abortions to pregnancies among African-Americans much lower.

62.   On those early attacks see Dula, in this volume; Angela Y. Davis, *Women, Race and Class* (New York: Random House, 1981). Nat Henthoff has often delineated the new eugenics argument. See, for example, his "Abortion as Population Control," *Washington Post*, July 29, 1989, A17, and "Abortion and the Specter of Pro-Choice Eugenics," *Washington Post*, May 25, 1991, A31. In the former, Henthoff pointedly quotes Jesse Jackson's eloquent warning that the arguments for abortion (and for abortion-rights) that appeal to the social costs of additional people tend to provide justification as well for "killing other forms of incompleteness . . . crippleness [sic], old age." Indeed, Henthoff cites Molly Yard's appeal to the costs to the planet of carrying further population and to admonitions of the politician Geraldine Ferraro and journalist Ken Auletta, suggesting that legally restricting abortions would result in more criminals and welfare mothers. As Henthoff observes, this marks a shift in the strategy of those in the American debate who wish to insure easily-and cheaply-available abortion. Whereas formerly they appealed to the importance of safeguarding the privacy-rights of women, today they follow the line of earlier eugenicists in defending easy abortion for the good of the planet, the society, and the race. In "Abortion and the Specter of Pro-Choice Eugenics," he discusses the assessment of the physically challenged implicit in such legislation as that recently passed in Maryland prohibiting any interference with a woman's decision to abort a fetus with any "serious" defect, deformity, or abnormality.

63.   Sanders, in this volume.

64.   Ibid.

65.   Ibid., (emphasis added).

66.   Stanley Crouch, *Notes of a Hanging Judge*, 101; cf. Shelby Steele, *The Content of Our Character*, 160. Clarence Thomas, a black judge whose conservative political views place him much further from the mainstream of African-American thought than Crouch, eloquently makes the same point with less hostility but equal passion.

"There seems to be an obsession with painting blacks as an unthinking group of automatons, with a common set of views, opinions, and ideas. Anyone who . . . disagrees with the 'black viewpoint' is immediately cast as . . . some sort of anti-black renegade. . . . Many of us accept the mockery and ostracism in order to have our own ideas, which are not intended to coincide with anyone else's. . . . The popularity of our ideas is unimportant, hence, polls and referendums are not needed to sustain or clarify them. . . . We certainly cannot claim to have progressed much in this country as long as it is insisted that our intellects are controlled entirely by our pigmentation, with its countless variations, even though our individual experiences are entirely different" (Quoted in "Clarence Thomas in his Own Words," *New York Times* July 2, 1991, A14). Of course, Thomas's reference to pigmentation is a straw man, but his point about the diversity of individual experience suffices to undermine even the more plausible view that it is the shared African-American historical experience that should determine our ideas.

67.   Leonard Harris, *Philosophy Born of Struggle*, xv.

68.   Sartre, in *Orphee Noir*, described the heightened African self-consciousness of the negritude movement in Hegelian terms, that is, as an antithesis set against the thesis of white racism. As such, it could serve only to "prepare the synthesis or realization of the human in a society without races. Thus negritude is the root of its own destruction, it is a transition and not a conclusion, a means and not an ultimate end" (quoted by Frantz Fanon in "The Fact of Blackness," 120).

69.   See the discussion on Bobby Seale's admission that the Black Panthers' distributed Little Red Books without reading them in the *New York Times* September 9, 1990, Sec. 2, p. 22

70.   See the controversy over Shelby Steele in the *Washington Post*, October 10, 1990, D1-2.

71.   Shelby Steele, *The Content of Our Character*, 100.

72.   Ibid., 72.

73.   Charles Johnson, *Being and Race*, 120.

74.   Ibid., 29.

75.   Murray proposes that the African-American "concept of self is equated with that of 'community,'" but it is not easy to see how to take this. If it were meant literally, then there could be no divergence between self-interest and communal interest (see "Minority Perspectives," 10).

Steele writes of a young man, "race was the ultimate arbiter of his individuality not because, I believe, he was so loyal to his race, but because race excused his fears. Racial identity is a necessary element in the overall identity of any black, but when we *use* it to recompose our fears, we always suppress our individuality and create a distorted view of ourselves and the world" (Steele, *The Content of Our Character*, 70). Steele explains (p. 58) that by "recomposition" he means a psychological defense in which we re-interpret and distort a situation as a way of legitimizing to ourselves the replacement of some painful emotional reaction we have had to the situation (such as shame) with a more bearable one (for example, resentment). One quibble with Steele: where he speaks of "identity," I think it best to speak of "self-image" lest we confuse the objective metaphysical question of who one is with the subjective conceptual question of how one thinks of oneself. I think Kwame Anthony Appiah's use of the term "ethical identity" for something like the latter betrays just this confusion (see his "'But Would That Still Be Me?' Notes on Gender, 'Race,' Ethnicity, as Sources of 'Identity,'" *Journal of Philosophy*, vol. 87, No. 10 (October, 1990): 493-499).

76. Kwame Anthony Appiah, "The Conservation of 'Race,'" *Black American Literature Forum* 23 (1989): 55. He defines "extrinsic racists" as people who "make moral distinctions between members of different races, because they believe that the racial essence entails certain morally relevant qualities" (p. 44).

77. I recently saw a sign exhorting us to pursue the values of "African consciousness," among which values were listed both creativity (*kuumba*) and unity (*umoja*). Perhaps one way of putting the point I am making here is that we must recognize the tension between creativity and unity of thought (at least, insofar as the latter requires ideological uniformity).

78. Shelby Steele thinks black people emphasize victimization by whites in a bid for the sort of moral power that comes from being innocent. "This . . . innocence gave blacks their first real power in American life—victimization metamorphosed into power via innocence" (Steele, *The Content of Our Character*, 14). Dinesh D'Souza raises the deeper question: why is being a victim something people in American cultures dwell on and allow to shape their self-image? After all, the victim is the loser, and in many cultures this might be deemed something ignoble and shameful. Recall Nietzsche's self-consciously post-Christian derision of what he saw as the Jews' claim to find in their history of defeats the story of God's chosen people. The case of Nietzsche might indicate that Christianity plays a crucial role in the elevation of the victim in Western culture, and this, in fact, is D'Souza's own view (Dinesh D'Souza, *Illiberal Education*, 302).

79. A similar problem may distort African-American fiction. Charles Johnson writes: "Black fiction comprises, one must confess, an overwhelmingly tragic literature. It is full of failures . . . . Whites in this history act; blacks can only *react*" (*Being and Race*, 7).

80. Immanuel Kant, *Critique of Practical Reason and Other Writings in Moral Philosophy*, tr. Lewis White Beck (New York: Garland Publishing, 1976).

81. Martin Peretz discusses the debasement of the term "community" in "Word Games," *New Republic* (November 5, 1990), 46. His harsh judgment is that "the black populace of our country is not really a community. . . ." Though he immediately adds the comparative, "any more than the white populace is," it is clear that Peretz's view is that much of the black populace is *further* removed from true community. He makes a strong case. "Community is the home of morality," he writes, adding that "community doesn't exist, except as a slogan, where family has been eroded. The family provides us with the first paradigm of authority. Without authority there is

no structure, no obligation, no responsibility. And this increasingly is what
obtains among the black poor."

  82.   As being an African-American is not sufficient for membership in
the community, neither is it necessary. People of many races may be members of a community if they are promoting its common good. This openness
is true even of a community that is an African-American community in fact,
by virtue of its numerically predominant racial group, or the source of its vision of the good life people.

  83.   See Raymond Williams, *Keywords.*

  84.   See the historical essay on the term "Culture" in Raymond Williams, *Keywords*, 87-93; and, in the same volume, the essay on "Civilization,"
57-60. Note that these definitions also make intelligible the notions of the cultured (that is, cultivated) individual and "high culture." Indeed, multiculturalism becomes interesting and plausible when it is taken as the thesis that
there are many avenues, found in diverse groups, along which someone may
develop in genuinely human ways. In contrast, he theses sometimes advanced by self-proclaimed "multiculturalists,"e.g., that every group's "way
of life" has produced great works or, more strongly, is worthy of *equal* consideration, seem quite implausible and extravagant.

  85.   Predictably, according to journalistic reports, there are social scientists at work trying to show that even unwed pregnancy among teenagers is
a "rational" response to their situation without dire financial or health risks.
Ann Hulbert exposes what appear to be serious flaws in this research ("Poor
Conceptions," *New Republic*, November 12, 1990: 21-23). See also the ensuing
correspondence between Ms. Hulbert and Professor Arline Geronimus, one
of the researchers whose work she criticizes, in *New Republic*, December 24,
1990: 2, 42.

  Louis Sullivan, the Secretary of Health and Human Services and himself
a black man, takes a more sober view of the sorry "way of life" of too many
young African-Americans. Among his sound recommendations are these:
"We must emphasize character [which is] the capacity to forego short-run
personal gratification in order to achieve long-term accomplishment. . . . We
must maintain and strengthen families [against social and "cultural" forces
tending to discourage marriage, and to encourage divorce, abandonment,
out-of-wedlock births, and child-neglect]" (see Louis Sullivan, "Without
Hope or Humanity," *Washington Post*, January 6, 1991, C7.

  According to an earlier magazine article, the writer Toni Morrison has
praised teenagers who become pregnant for following the hand of "Nature"
("The Toni Award," *The New Republic*, June 19, 1989: 9-10). This remark says
something about what happens when people appeal to nature for normative
guidance in an intellectual climate entirely cut off from the natural law philosophical tradition.

  The journalist Morton Kondracke identifies three leading schools of
thought among students of the contemporary problems confronting African-
Americans: the first emphasizes current and residual racism; the second,

economic needs; the third, the failure of institutions to inculcate virtues important for success. I have here drawn attention to the concerns stressed by this last school but, as Kondracke himself notes, there is no reason to think that when we draw attention to one set of contributing factors we imply that the others are insignificant (Morton Kondracke, "The Two Black Americas," *New Republic*, February 6, 1989, 17-20).

86. Gates writes that the "strategy" behind Two Live Crew's sexual braggadocio in their controversial recording "Nasty As They Wanna Be" is to take "racist stereotypes about black sexuality" and to "explode [them] with exaggeration." His discussion ties the group's lyrics to the "street culture" tradition called "playing the dozens." Though many of the album's songs are both misogynist in content and obscene in expression, this is the closest Professor Gates can bring himself to condemnation: "Much more troubling than [their] so-called obscenity is the group's overt sexism. . . . We must not allow ourselves to sentimentalize street culture: the appreciation of verbal virtuosity does not lessen one's obligation to critique bigotry in all its pernicious forms" (H. L. Gates, "Two Live Crew, Decoded," *New York Times*, June 19, 1990: A23.

87. "It is a peculiar sensation, this double-consciousness . . . one ever feels his twoness—an American, a Negro; two souls, two thoughts, two unreconciled strivings; two warring ideals in one dark body, whose dogged strength alone keeps it from being torn asunder.

"The history of the Negro in America is the history of this strife—this longing to . . . merge his double self into a better and truer self. In this merging he wishes neither of the older selves to be lost.

". . . He simply wishes to make it possible for a man to be both a Negro and an American (W. E. B. DuBois, *The Souls of Black Folk* [Millwood, New York: Kraus-Thomson, 1973], 3-4).

88. "Making the African connection, rejoining roots, and building common bonds have carried far more weight among African-American scholars than severing roots or decrying cultural heritage. The cultural roots more likely disdained are those festered by the corrupting and deprivational circumstances of slavery and racism" (Leonard Harris, *Philosophy Born of Struggle*, xv). Harris doesn't tell us just how to interpret this statement. My point, however, is that to see *everything* American about African-Americans as festered by racism is both to deform our experience on this continent and to blind oneself to the unique opportunities our position here affords us. It is also, of course, a prescription for permanent self-hatred.

89. Kwame Anthony Appiah, "Conservation of 'Race,'" 47.

90. I don't wish to endorse the "End of History" triumphalism that James E. Bowman repudiates in "The Plight of Poor African-Americans" (pp. 173-187). The struggle for liberal constitutional democracy is not yet over, for predicaments such as those posed by homelessness and poverty still jeopardize democracies from within. Moreover, even if we accept the unduly optimistic judgment that Marxism is no longer a threat to free and just social

orders, having been destroyed by its own internal intellectual and social contradictions, its "specter," in Marx's prescient image, may haunt our politics for some time to come.

Professor Cone may be an example of someone whose thinking has moved in what I take to be the wrong direction. In a new preface to his influential 1970 book *A Black Theology of Liberation*, Cone repents his failure twenty years ago to tie the "black power" struggle to "Third World" liberation movements, to link racism to economic exploitation, and to divorce himself more fully than he did from what he sometimes calls "white theology" (see James H. Cone, *A Black Theology of Liberation*, 2nd ed. [Maryknoll, New York: Orbis, 1986], xiii-xxii).

Throughout this preface, one looks in vain for any indication that Professor Cone regrets having used language that degraded the moral crusade to secure our constitutional and moral rights into a mere power struggle between the races; that he recognizes the extent to which the liberation of the less-developed countries is today best represented in the anticommunist works of Fang Lizhi and Mrs. Chammorro, in the drive to transform such nations as post-Nyerere Tanzania into multiparty states, and, perhaps, in the counsel of Vargas Llosa and others that the free-market be used to restructure Latin American economies; that he has had second thoughts about the crudity of reducing the task of approaching the study of God from a perspective whose sources include the experiences of black people to a senseless opposition of "black theology" to "white theology." (On some moral differences between the civil rights and black power movements, see Shelby Steele, *The Content of Our Character*, chap. 4, and Stanley Crouch, *Notes of a Hanging Judge*, chap. 2).

91.   Charles Johnson, *Being and Race*, 123.

92.   The question of how to assimilate our past is a principal theme powerfully developed in August Wilson's play, *The Piano Lesson* (New York: Dutton, 1990). In the drama, a family must decide what to do with an old piano for which an ancestor was sold and into which have been carved scenes depicting the family's history. Should it be sold for money and the money used to purchase the farm on which their forebears had been enslaved? Or should it remain in the house where it is unplayed, save for the young daughter's lessons? What is the best use of the old instrument today: to be played, sold, or learned from?

93.   Cited in Cheryl Sanders, "Problems and Limitations," in this volume. Sartre wrote, "The Negro, as we have said, creates an 'anti-racist racism' for himself" (see Frantz Fanon, "The Fact of Blackness," p. 120). Kwame Anthony Appiah finds an element of this in some of the race-pride literature issuing from this black awareness and, while unconvinced by Sartre's claim that this is a necessary stage, calls for the transcendence that Sartre predicted of such racism (see Kwame Anthony Appiah, "The Conservation of 'Race,'" p. 58n9).

TOM L. BEAUCHAMP:

Response to Jorge Garcia

Four issues arise from Professor Garcia's paper: (1) different types of relativism and their defensibility; (2) interpretations that Garcia does and does not defend or commit himself to; (3) some conceptual problems about the English-language term "moral"; and (4) the question, "Are African-American Perspectives Unique?"

TYPES OF RELATIVISM

Garcia is suspicious of theses in support of moral relativism based on cultural relativity. So am I. Many notions, however, are subsumed under the rubric of relativism, and we should take care to specify the relativism or relativisms that are at stake. I begin, then, by distinguishing different types of relativism.

First, it is a mistake to formulate problems of moral and social relativism so that cultural relativism, that is, diversity of belief deriving from cultural diversity, is the important or even major form of relativism. Diversity of moral belief may exist within a *single* culture at any point in its history. Moreover, culture may not even be the relevant source of conflicting beliefs. As an accident of history, it is irrelevant to the question of *moral* relativism. Though we tend to be most sensitive to issues of relativity because of what we take to be cultural differences, relativity based on individual, national, or political differences may be far more important than cultural roots of relativity. And even if the roots of relativism are cultural, it does not follow that they are ethnic roots.

Second, an important distinction that Garcia largely brushes aside is that between a *relativism of standards* and a *relativism of judgments*. By "standards" I mean foundational moral values or principles on the basis of which moral judgments are made; by "judgments" I mean acts of evaluating in which moral values or principles are clarified, specified, applied, or interpreted. A principle of respect for the autonomy of persons is a standard in this sense. A judgment that we should allow mental patients to refuse drug treatments is a judgment that may appeal for justification to the principle of respect for autonomy.

Garcia appears to have directed his arguments largely to a relativism of standards. Relativism of judgments is, however, pervasive in human social life, and most of the real problems about relativism center on a relativity of judgment, not on a relativism of standards. For example, you and I may disagree with Edmund Pellegrino's judgment that physicians may never with moral justification take the life of any patient. Inspection of our viewpoints indicates, however, that we do not disagree with him on the foundational moral principles of killing, medical beneficence, or patient autonomy. Instead, differences on entirely other matters affect our moral judgments. We may disagree, say, in our predictions about the social consequences of physician-induced killing, or we may have different appraisals of whether physicians can ever be sure that they have understood the patient's judgments and deepest wishes.

In a context of pluralism, we cannot reasonably expect to agree in our judgments about the moral acceptability of such matters as (1) reverse discrimination; (2) the conditions, if any, under which abortion is warranted; (3) whether the "ethics of trust" should be allowed to define physician-patient relationships; (4) whether national health insurance should be provided to all citizens; (5) whether the mentally disturbed should be committed without their consent; or (6) whether civil disobedience is ever justified. In our disagreements we often affirm the same basic principles or values (the sanctity of life; respect for individual choice; the value of the family) despite our different conclusions, positions, or judgments.

Our conflicting judgments in these affairs are rarely, if ever, based on different moral principles or foundational standards. The problem is more likely to be that we specify, adapt, or otherwise apply or use the same principles in different ways. Or, in a circumstance of conflict between principles, we may weigh them differently; that is, we may attach different moral weights to the same (nonrelative) moral principles. These are distinct and massive problems of relativity of judgment; however, they do not necessarily involve a relativity of standards or foundational principles.[1]

It looks at one point as if Garcia implicitly recognizes and accepts this distinction between a relativism of judgments and a relativism of standards. He says, "Nor will it do for [the cultural relativist] to say that [some] judgments differ from ours in content but are similar in the rationale supporting them, for this will tend to mean that the relativism evaporates as we approach the deeper moral claims that serve as the epistemic or justificatory basis of our judgments or practices."[2]

This observation is correct, but Garcia seems to conclude from it that relativism in general evaporates under the pressure of this argument. I reach the more qualified conclusion that although a relativism of standards is certainly put under pressure by the argument, a relativism of judgments is actually presupposed by the argument. Since I think relativism of judgments is the more difficult problem, both practically and philosophically, I will remain unsatisfied until this problem is treated.

GARCIA'S RELATIVITY THESIS

When I initially read Garcia's paper, I thought he was rejecting a relativism of standards and had no position on a relativism of judgments. On second and third readings, however, I abandoned this interpretation. I began to wonder whether he rejects *any* form of relativism. His strongest comment seems to be that "there are serious problems confronting any form of cultural relativism that is significantly extensive, deep, or strong in its judgmental scope."[3] This is not tantamount to a rejection of any form of relativism, or even to a reprimand.

My current interpretation of Garcia's argument differs considerably from my original reading. I interpret the paper as follows: In *accepting* Banner's thesis that there is an extramental and extrapersonal order of things, Garcia means concomitantly to reject a (cultural) relativism of standards; but in *rejecting* Banner's second thesis that perspective has no application in ethics, he allows for "the existence and legitimacy of differing perspectives in ethics, even differing ethnic perspectives in ethics."[4] He thereby implicitly accepts a relativism of judgment. An ethnic perspective in conflict with some competing perspective is in his analysis a relativism of judgment.

Garcia has defined a "relativity thesis" only as "holding that *some* moral judgments are *somehow* relative to the codes or lifestyles of cultural groups" (my italics).[5] My interpretation of his relativism is consistent with this definition, but I leave open how extensive, deep, and strong his commitment to relativism is. I believe he makes no clear statement on this question.

If my interpretation of Garcia's position is correct, I agree with it, just as I agree with many of his other views on these problems. I agree, that one cannot smuggle in some principle of tolerance and still be a strong relativist (since tolerance is, on relativistic grounds, nothing more than another local value), and I agree that the concept of morality places constraints on what can count as a moral form of relativism.[6]

My interpretation of Garcia, as a relativist of a certain sort, is entirely compatible with his insistence that different standpoints or perspectives may provide us with a better understanding of how things objectively ought to be.[7] All forms of (descriptive) relativism are compatible with all forms of how things ought objectively to be (normative objectivity). This is one reason why philosophers have typically judged cultural relativism to be irrelevant to normative moral theory.

One caution is in order, however, about how much tolerance a relativism of judgment should encourage and permit. No general theory of an *acceptable* relativism suggests that we must tolerate *all* acts of others, including those that violate the (nonrelative, foundational) standards of morality. Accordingly, at least some judgments allegedly constituting moral views will turn out to be morally unacceptable, and may be recognized as such, without inconsistency, by one who accepts a relativism of judgments (although not by one who accepts a relativism of standards).

Such a relativism of judgments is, however, a difficult claim to fulfill, for reasons I want now to discuss.

THE CONCEPT OF MORALITY

Garcia notes the importance for a moral relativist of showing that alleged moral conflicts are really moral. If one of the conflicting judgments is not moral, then we do not have moral relativism, even if we have some form of relativism. Garcia then observes that moral judgments are recognizable as moral only "insofar as they pertinently resemble what we ordinarily call moral."[8] He notes that although he may be charged with a kind of conceptual Eurocentrism, we need to begin from where we are, which is with "the moral" as reflected in the English language.

This argument may not get at the deeper problems that may, at least in part, underlie the accusation of Eurocentrism that Garcia is trying to shake off. These problems concern the criteria that govern the use of the term "moral" in the English language. In recent philo-

sophical literature on the meaning of "moral," analysis of the concept
has been provided in terms of such "marks of the moral" as prescrip-
tivity, universalizability, overridingness, and the promotion of
human welfare. Each of these criteria has come under attack (as neither necessary or sufficient for making a judgment or principle
"moral"). It could be argued that these and other candidates for criteria of the moral are not necessary or essential conditions of morality,
although each may be *relevant* in mapping the geography of morality.
That is, each may be a mark that identifies some criterion of the
moral, though not an essential mark.

Let's assume that the full geography of the concept of morality is
muddy and complicated, because morality has been shaped by law,
ethnic communities, religion, government, and other social institutions—all of which use general action-guides to prescribe behavior.
This assumption suggests the need for a discussion of whether the
term "morality" would be better understood as a *diverse set of relevant*
conditions (or marks) than as a *set of necessary and sufficient* conditions.

The hypothesis is relevant to our discussion in the following way:
If morality is a sufficiently open-textured concept, so that one can *correctly* judge two or more conflicting judgments to be moral when the
conflicting judgments call on (partially or wholly) different criteria of
the moral, then we have a deep problem of conceptual relativism.
The suggestion here is that the English term "moral" is not univocal
but has the character of what is sometimes called a family resemblance concept: "Morality" cannot be given any single, exhaustive
definition or analysis in terms of criteria, conditions, or marks of the
moral, because there are too many senses of the "moral"—or at least
too many diverse marks or criteria that can be used to classify judgments or actions as moral. Garcia's appeal to the English term
"moral" as a bulwark against relativism might then lose much of its
force.

If this analysis is accepted, morality as identified by the English
term "moral" is not one thing but many things in combination. Because only some of the several criteria making up the concept must
be present on any given occasion, there can be different senses of
morality (a distinction implied by the terms "moral," and "ethics"):
e.g., theological ethics; professional ethics; the ethics of ethnic perspectives; personal ethics. What makes physician confidentiality a
moral matter may, on this analysis, be very different from the criteria
that make the Watergate scandal, euthanasia, or polygamy moral
matters. Yet each of these is a genuinely moral problem.

THE REALITY OF UNIQUE
AFRICAN-AMERICAN PERSPECTIVES

The word "ethnos" originally referred to a nation or people, but we have come to use the derivative term "ethnic" largely for racial or minority groups. "Ethnic perspectives," I suggest, may not be the best way to represent or defend the views for which Garcia argues. Ethnic histories may generate or reinforce a certain moral viewpoint, and we may value an ethnic heritage for this contribution. But there is nothing particularly *ethnic* about any of the seven "African-American Ethical Perspectives" specifically discussed in Garcia's paper.[9] Nor is there anything distinctively African-American about them; Native Americans may well be as disposed to them as African-Americans. Just as the moral perspectives put forward by feminists are not always unique to women, so many African-American perspectives may not be unique to African-Americans.

This observation leads to further questions about the topic of this conference as a whole. Anything constituting an "African-American Perspective on Biomedical Ethics" (of the sort mentioned by Garcia) is only contingently and historically associated with any particular ethnic group; had history been different, that same perspective might have constituted not an African-American perspective but some other group's perspective, and not necessarily an ethnic group at that.

NOTES

1. Different persons often give different meanings to central terms, principles, and values invoked in such circumstances of disagreement. If, however, the meanings are changed, it is reasonable to conclude that the standards are relative, not merely the judgments.

2. Jorge Garcia, "African-American Perspectives, Cultural Relativism, and Normative Issues: Some Conceptual Questions," in this volume.

3. Ibid.

4. Ibid.

5. Ibid.

6. The relativist cannot hold that a principle of tolerance is demanded by morality itself, because this appeal is nonrelativistic. It also opens the door to other nonrelativistic standards. Indeed, we may suspect that something like a universal principle of respect for persons underlies and gives moral force to, the normative relativists' appeal for tolerance and respect. A

moral principle of tolerance of other practices and beliefs lead inexorably to the abandonment of relativism.

7.   Jorge Garcia, "African-American Perspectives," in this volume.

8.   Ibid.

9.   Ibid.

WILLIAM A. BANNER:

Response to Jorge Garcia

I shall concern myself with three matters that are discussed in Professor Garcia's paper, namely, the notion of "perspective," the idea of one moral community, and the thesis of "cultural relativism."

PERSPECTIVE

On the matter of "perspective," my position in the paper to which Professor Garcia refers rejects the notion of "ethnic perspective," not the notion of perspective as such.[1] There is a realm of experience in which I consider it correct to speak of "perspective," namely, the realm of sense awareness or sense perception. It may be helpful here to say a word or two about sense perception. G. E. Moore, in an essay entitled, "The Status of Sense-Data," distinguishes five classes of what he calls "sensory experiences," namely, images, dreams, hallucinations and certain illusory experiences, after-images, and *sensations* proper, i.e., direct sensory apprehension or reception.[2]

It is the last of these, namely, sensations proper, that may be taken (sometimes at least) to be the awareness of physical or material objects. That our *direct* sense knowledge is of sense data and not of objects as John Locke maintained and that there may be sense data that are not parts of the surfaces of objects, as H. H. Price maintained are matters of debate that I will pass over at this time.[3]

I wish to affirm for myself the common sense view that sense knowledge is of objects. And to this must be added the view that sense awareness, notably visual sensation, is *perspectival*. What I

74

perceive is what is present to my sense as the concrete and particular object under the precise spatio-temporal conditions of the situation in which I am a percipient. The "perspectives" of sense knowledge are individual and perhaps *private*, in as much as sensations and images cannot be shared. My distinct visual awareness of a colored object is simply mine.

At the same time, perspectives are *public*, insofar as an object would present the same appearance as *datum* to anyone who senses or sees it from the same point of space and under the same conditions of observation as I do. There is indeed an interchangeability of viewing or perspective among observers both at the level of common sense and in descriptive science. I will leave aside for the present the variations in sense awareness arising presumably from an aberration, in or derangement of, a sense organ, as in color blindness and in persons suffering from jaundice.

As one moves from the particularity of sense knowledge to the level of thinking, the cognitive landscape is different. At the level of concepts, it seems that one would not speak in a strict way of "perspective" or "perspectives." There are no spatio-temporal determinants from which an individual thinks. For a problem or subject matter, there is simply the *statement of the question* (after the fashion proposed by Descartes in Part II of the *Discourse on Method*). There are no fixed conditions, affecting the mind, that set limits on what an individual thinks, whether the individual initiates an inquiry or investigation or responds to what has been initiated by another person. Analysis and discussion are *human* capabilities that are assisted toward actualization in a variety of ways, such as by parents and teachers, by the promptings of friendships, by the distinct stimulation of university life, by the broad intellectual climate, and by the direct or immediate situation of pressing problems and dilemmas.

Professor Garcia recognizes, as I do, the appropriateness or appositeness of an individual's engagement with one problem rather than another in a given social context or situation, particularly where this problem is very serious and has been either ignored or inadequately addressed. But this condition does not require or entail in any way an "ethnic perspective," either on the part of the individual who initiates the investigation of the particular problem or on the part of those who respond to what has been initiated. If a genuine problem exists and a case can be made for its solution, the whole matter is necessarily addressed to all members of the scientific and moral community.

That some Europeans or persons of European background have confined their thinking and acting to the pursuits and problems of persons and groups in their immediate social and cultural milieu and have ignored, trivialized, or distorted the pursuits and problems of other groups does not reveal, in the realm of analysis, a European "perspective" or "frame of mind." What is dealt with in investigation is done either adequately or inadequately, rigorously or not; and to ignore, trivialize, or distort matters that pertain to what one proposes to examine is to go about the task inadequately. One can dispose of shoddy scholarship without involving the idea of "ethnic perspective," thus avoiding the undesirable possibility that every critique will be turned into an ad hominem attack of one ethnic group on another.

It is expected that every investigation will meet the demands of fidelity to matters of fact and fidelity to the universal rules of logic. In a democracy, and especially in academic and professional circles, there is the additional expectation that every debatable matter will be aired and examined in every possible forum or seminar. The importance of these expectations is persuasive: one thinks of an investigator or a *protagonist* in his own society who wishes, *as a citizen*, to make claims on the resources of the whole society for the solution of the problem at hand.

COMMUNITY

The question is properly raised concerning the idea of *one moral community*, an idea that Professor Garcia regards as so broad as to be empty or virtually empty, indeed the idea of a community that does not exist. There are, of course, existing social units of greater or lesser extensity that can be taken as existing moral communities. One recognizes that every individual is a member of many social units, from the family to the state, in which certain affinities are acknowledged and either certain practices are observed according to rules of conduct, or there is the expectation that certain practices will be observed. Every social unit is thus governed by practices or customs that constitute the ethos or pattern of the group's life. These observations are made, however, on the level of sociology or social anthropology, not on the level of ethics or moral philosophy.

One must say that prevailing practice is simply prevailing practice and not *morality* unless this practice (together with its underlying rules) embraces the claim or claims of the individual on a certain *quality* of life. The interests or claims or *rights* of the individual are therefore distinguishable from what is approved or commanded in his or her group. And it is in terms of such claims or rights that the practices and structures of the group are brought under *moral* scrutiny as supporting or opposing what is best for the individual. Morality emerges, as Socrates makes clear in Plato's *Apology*, from social-and self-examinations that project a certain *quality of life* (for the individual) as the criterion and goal of all deliberate behavior. Moral analysis thus provides the premise or premises for an ongoing debate concerning what precisely is good and right and just in any and every social context.

As David Hume discovered in his inquiries, a moral principle readily extends the commitment from mutual advantage in the family to mutual advantage in society as a whole and ultimately to mutual advantage in the interrelation between separate societies.[4] It would seem that when one talks about human advantage or human claims (or rights), one addresses *one* moral community, not many communities. One declares, in so many words, that the right of a child to adequate nutrition and health care in the immediate family is the same right of the same child outside the village or community, outside the region or province, indeed, even beyond the limits of society as a stranger or refugee in a foreign land.

Maurice Merleau-Ponty has said that through a deeper anthropological understanding we have come to see that the human being is eccentric to himself and that the social finds its center only in the individual human being.[5] Philosophy, he has also said, is "the consciousness we must maintain . . . of the open and successive community of [others] living, speaking, and thinking in one another's presence."[6] And, in still another place, he has said that in such a broadened consciousness "the frontiers between cultures are erased; for the first time, no doubt, a world civilization becomes the order of the day."[7]

RELATIVISM

Finally, on the matter of cultural relativism, I am in agreement with Professor Garcia in raising questions that I would word as follows:

1. Does cultural relativism involve some or all moral judgments, including judgments concerning justice?
2. Are diverse moral judgments the expression of diverse and compatible interests reconciled through the intermediation of reflection (as Ralph Barton Perry maintained) or expressions of diverse and incompatible interests both within and between cultures (as Max Weber contended)?

3. Can it be seriously maintained that so-called moral codes contain "ultimate ought statements" that cannot be appraised and ranked according to a transcultural norm or norms?

Cultural relativism arose in the ancient Western world apparently with the teaching of the Sophists. In the modern world, one thinks of Montesquieu's *Spirit of the Laws* as setting forth a cultural anthropology that embraces both historicism and relativism. There is, clearly, disagreement among relativists. One recognizes that it is one thing to argue simply for the appreciation of pluralism in life and style within a complex democratic society, in the fashion of Professor Alain Locke and quite another thing to maintain with Baron de Montesquieu that climate, soil, tradition, the structure of social institutions, and the historical laws of change produce the laws, manners, and customs of a society in accordance with necessary causation.[8] One can indeed subscribe to the relativism of Alain Locke without endorsing the relativism of Montesquieu. One wishes to say, in somewhat different words, that the recognition of relativity in normative judgments and in social practice does not require the adoption of a thoroughgoing relativism that reduces all moral judgment to the caprice of taste, time, and circumstance.

St. Augustine, in the third book of his *Confessions*, states the relation of the *variable* and the *invariant* in human affairs in these words:

> [It may be observed] in one [person], and in one day, and in one house, different things to be fit for different members, and one thing to be lawful now, which an hour hence is not so; and something to be permitted or commanded in one corner, which is forbidden and punishable in another. Is justice thereupon various or mutable? No; but the times, rather, which justice governs, are not like one another, for they are times.[9]

It is an invariant element of human life and human affairs that the thoroughgoing relativist fails to recognize or obscures while giving sustained attention to the descriptions of cultural diversity. This invariant element, it would seem, is affirmed in all statements or declarations of *human rights* and in all uncoerced support of these rights by diverse societies—within their precise borders and beyond.

NOTES

1. See my *Is There an African-American Perspective on Biomedical Ethics? The View from Philosophy*; a paper presented at the Georgetown University Conference on African-American Perspectives on Biomedical Ethics, November 1989 (in this volume).

2. G. E. Moore, *Philosophical Studies* (London: Routledge and Kegan Paul, 1922), 168.

3. John Locke, *An Essay Concerning Human Understanding*, (New York: Samuel Marken, 1825), 2:23; H. H. Price, *Perception*, 2nd ed. (London: Meuthen, 1964), chapter 5.

4. David Hume, *Enquiry Concerning the Principles of Morals*, I, 153.

5. Maurice Merleau-Ponty, *Signs*, (Evanston, Illinois: Northwestern University Press, 1964), 123.

6. Ibid., 110.

7. Ibid., 124.

8. Baron de Montesquieu, *Spirit of the Laws*, 1, 14-19.

9. *St. Augustine's Confessions*, trans. William Watts, in Loeb Classical Library, 26 (London: William Heinemann, Ltd., 1977), 125.

KWASI WIREDU

The Moral Foundations of
African Culture

In the strictest sense morality is universal, nay, *essential*, to human culture. Any society without at least a modicum of morality must collapse. But what is morality in this sense? It is the observance of rules for the harmonious adjustment of the individual's interests to those of others. This observance is, of course, a minimal concept of morality. A richer concept of morality, one more pertinent to human flourishing, will have an essential reference to that special kind of motivation called "the sense of duty." Morality in this sense involves not just the de facto conformity to the requirements of the harmony of interests, but a conformity to those requirements that is inspired by imaginative and sympathetic identification with the interests of others even at the cost of a possible abridgement of one's own interests. This requirement is not a demand for supererogatory altruism, but a minimum of altruism is essential to the moral motivation. In this sense, too, morality is probably universal to all human societies, if not to all individuals.

The foregoing reflection does not exclude the possibility of a legitimate basis for differentiating the morals of the various peoples of the world—for at least three reasons. First, although morality in the senses just discriminated is the same wherever and whenever it is practiced, different peoples, groups, and individuals understand morality in different ways. The contrasting moral standpoints of humanism and supernaturalism, for example, illustrate this diversity. Second, the concrete cultural context in which a moral principle is applied may give it a distinctive coloring. Third, and most important, there is a broader concept of morals closely continuous with this one in regard to which the contingencies of space, time, and climate play a constitutive role. This broader morality pertains to the domain called "custom," and includes such things as the prescriptions and proscriptions operative in a community regarding death, work and leisure, reward and retribution, aspirations and aversions, attitudes to pleasure and pain, and the relationships between the sexes, the generations, and other social categories and classes. The combined impact of such regulations about life and thought in a society provide a distinctive impression of its morals.

A HUMANISTIC ORIENTATION

I begin with the manner of conceiving morals. African moral conceptions seem generally to have a humanistic orientation. Competent anthropological studies lend substantial support to this claim. Nevertheless, anthropological accounts are not always philosophically inquisitive, and I prefer, in elaborating on this characterization, to rely on my own native knowledge of the life and thought of the Akans of Ghana. On this basis, I can affirm the humanism in question more uninhibitedly. The commonest formulation of this outlook is in the saying, which almost any Akan adult or even young hopeful will proffer on the slightest provocation, *onipa na ohia*: it is a human being that has value. The English translation of this saying, though pertinent, needs to be supplemented, for the crucial term here has a double connotation. The word "(o)hia" in this context means that which is valuable and needed. The first meaning imparts the message that all value derives from human interests; the second, that human fellowship is the most important of human needs. When fellowship is uppermost in consciousness, an Akan would be likely to elucidate the maxim to the effect that though you have all the gold in the world and a well-stocked wardrobe, if you were to call on these things in an hour of need, they would not respond; only a human being will respond: *Onipa ne asem; mefre sika a sika nnye so; mefre ntama a, ntama nnve so; onipa ne asem*. Already we see emerging the great stress on human sociality in Akan thought; before we pursue this angle, however, let me tarry awhile on the significance of Akan humanism.

An important implication of defining value in terms of human interests is the independence of morality from religion in the Akan outlook: what is good in general is what promotes human interests. Correspondingly, what is good in the more narrowly ethical sense is, by definition, what is conducive to the harmonization of those interests. Thus the will of God, not to talk of other extrahuman wills, is logically incapable of defining the good. On the Akan understanding of things, God is good in the highest; but God's goodness is conceptually the goodness of a just and benevolent ancestor, except that its quality and scale are assumed to be limitless. The prospect of punishment from God or some lesser being may concentrate the mind on the narrow path of virtue, but it does not create a sense of moral obligation, just as the probability of police intervention may conceivably give pause to a would-be burglar, though if he or she has any morals at all, it would not be thanks to the collective will of the police or the state.

This conceptual separation of morals from religion is responsible in some measure for the remarkable fact that there is no institutional religion in the Akan culture. The procedures associated with belief in sundry extrahuman beings of varying powers and inclinations, so often emphasized in accounts of African religions, are, in fact, practical utilitarian programs for tapping the resources of this world. The idea, in a nutshell, is that God fashioned out the cosmos with physical and quasi-physical, personal and quasi-personal potentialities, which human beings may bend to their purposes, if they learn how. Naturally, in dealing with beings and powers believed to be of a quasi-personal character, certain aspects of their behavior patterns will manifest important analogies to ordinary human interactions. For example, if one wants something from a being of supernatural repute who is open to persuasion mixed with praise, common sense is enough to recommend that one adopt an attitude of respect and circumspection toward that being and address it in a language of laudatory circumlocution reminiscent of worship. At the same time, one's calculative and utilitarian purpose belies any attribution of a specifically religious motivation. In fact, the Akans are known to be sharply contemptuous of "gods" who fail to deliver; continued respect is conditional on high scoring by the Akan reckoning.

In total contrast to the foregoing, the Akan attitude to the Supreme Being is one of unconditional reverence and absolute trust. Absent here is any notion that so perfect a being requires or welcomes institutions for singing or reciting its praises. Nor, relatedly, are any such institutions felt to be necessary for the dissemination of moral education or the reinforcement of the will to virtue.

The theater of moral upbringing is the home, at parents' feet and within range of input from one's kin. The mechanism is precept, example, correction; and the process is life-long. Although upbringing belongs to the beginning of our earthly careers, the need for correction is an unending contingency in mortal lives. As opposed to earlier stages in life, moral correction in adulthood, involves discourses of a high level and may entail the imposition of compensatory obligations, but at all stages verbal lessons in morality are grounded in conceptual and empirical considerations about human well being. On this basis the term "humanistic" is an apt characteristic of Akan moral thinking. And for the same reason, it is correct to describe that ethic as "nonsupernaturalistic" notwithstanding the Akans' sincere belief in a Supreme Being.

Insofar, then, as the concept of religion is applicable to the Akan outlook on life and reality, it can only refer to belief and trust in the Supreme Being. In this respect, Akan religion is purely intellectual. In this respect too, it is purely personal, being just a tenet of an individual's voluntary metaphysics, devoid of social entanglements. In truth, most Akans espouse this metaphysics as a matter of course. Akan conventional wisdom actually holds that the existence of God is so obvious it does not need to be taught even to a child: *Obi nkvere ak-wadaa Nyame*. Nevertheless, skeptics are not unknown in Akan society and a time-honored policy of peaceful laissez faire extends to them as to all others in matters of private persuasion.

Akan morality is also intellectual. Concrete moral situations are frequently highly composite tangles of imponderables; perceiving them in real life in their true lineaments is a cognitive accomplishment in itself. So too is the sure grasp of first principles and their judicious application to the particulars of conduct. Morality is also personal, for in the last analysis the individual must take responsibility for his or her own actions. But morality is, surely, neither purely intellectual, for it unquestionably has an irreducibly passionate ingredient, nor purely personal, for it is quintessentially social.

PERSONAL AND SOCIAL RESPONSIBILITIES

These insights are encapsulated in various Akan maxims and turns of phrase. Recognition of the intellectual dimension of right conduct is evident in the Akan description of a person of ethical maturity: *ob-dawenma*, one possessed of high thinking powers. Literally it says, "child, thinking child." It names one, in other words, as a thinking child of the species. The Akans are no less emphatic in their articulation of a sense of individual responsibility. According to a very popular proverb, it is because God dislikes injustice that God gave all people their own names (thereby forestalling any misattribution of responsibility). Along with this clear sense of individual responsibility comes an equally strong sense of the social reverberations of an individual's conduct. The primary responsibility for an action, positive or negative, rests with the doer, but a nontrivial, secondary responsibility extends to the individual's family and, in some cases, to the surrounding community.

For the Akans, therefore, a person is social not only because he or she lives in a community (the only context in which full, human development is possible), but also because, by internal constitution, a human being is part of a social whole.

The underlying doctrine is this. A person consists of three elements. One of these comes directly from God and is, in fact, a speck of divine substance. This element is the life principle in virtue of which all human beings are one; all are members of the universal family of humankind whose head and spring is God: *Nipa nyinaa ye Nyame mma; obiara nye asaase ba.* Literally, all human beings are children of God; not children of the earth. The two remaining elements are more mundane in origin. One, called "the blood principle," derives from the mother; the other, which we will call "the charisma principle," comes from the father.

The blood from the mother principally gives life to a person's body, while biological input from the father is responsible for the degree of personal presence that each individual subsequently develops at appropriate stages. (This input I take license to call the individual's "degree of charisma.") The ontological classification of these elements is not exactly straightforward. Suffice it to say that a dichotomy between the physical and the spiritual is unlikely to be a source of light in this connection. In any case, our interest is in the social significance of those components.

Both the maternal and paternal contributions to the person are bases of membership in specific social units. Akans are matrilineal; therefore, the blood principle situates a person in the important kinship units, namely, the lineage or, more extensively, the clan. Through the charisma principle one belongs to a grouping on the father's side that is largely ceremonial but also a framework for much goodwill.

The point now is this: on Akan showing, a person has a well-structured social identity even before birth. Thus, the Akan maxim that a human being descends from on high and alights in a town, *Se onipa siane fi soro a obesi kuro mu*, is an affirmation of his or her prior and well-defined social affiliations. But society presupposes rule—and moral rules, most essentially. Since all rules have their rationales, the ethical imagination, especially one thoroughly impregnated with visions of the ineluctable sociality of human existence, is challenged to discover the rationale of moral rules.

Among the Akans profound philosophic conceptions are frequently expressed by way of art motifs, and a celebrated answer to the ethical question is the image of a crocodile with one stomach and two heads locked in combat. The lesson? Although human beings have a core of common interests, they also have conflicting interests that precipitate real struggles; the aim of morality and, derivatively, of statesmanship, is to harmonize conflicting interests through systematic adjustment and adaptation. The one stomach symbolizes not only the commonality of interests but also a natural basis for possible solutions to the existential antinomy.

Two levels of solution to such conflicts are distinguishable, corresponding to a distinction foreshadowed in our opening paragraph: a level of prudence or enlightened self-interest, and a level of pure moral motivation. Both species of thought and intention may be equally adapted to securing the social good; the first through cool and calm ratiocination, the second through rational reflection and human sympathy. But they evoke different appraisals from people of goodwill. There will always be something unlovable about correctness of conduct bereft of passion. A Ghanaian comedian puts it even more strongly. Speaking in a deliberately unidiomatic bombast, he reflects; "Ability without sentimentality is nothing short of barbarity."

It appears, in fact, that teachers of morals everywhere have tended to find prudential considerations more psychologically efficacious in moral persuasion than abstract appeals to the goodwill. Certainly, Akan ethical reflection does not remain immobile at this level, but Akan discourse abounds in prudential maxims. Here are a few.

1. If you do not allow your neighbor to reach nine, you will never reach ten. (*Woamma wo yonko antwa nkronhg a worentwa edu.*)
2. Somebody's troubles have arrived; those of another are on the way. (*Obi de aba; obi de nam kwan so.*)
3. It is a fool that says, "My neighbor is the butt of the attack, not me." (*Kwasea na ose, "Ye de menyonko, yenne me."*)
4. The stick that was used to beat Takyi is the same that will be used to beat Nyankomago. (*Abaa a yede boo Takyi no aa na ye de bebo Nyankomago.*
5. One person's path will intersect with another's before too long. (*Obi kwan nkye na asi obi de mu.*)

That Akan ethics transcends this level of moral understanding is evident from other moral sayings. But I am commenting on one particularly instructive form of moral discourse. To a person whose conduct betrays obliviousness to the interests of others, we say, *Etua woyonko ho a etua dua mu*: "Sticking into your neighbor's flesh, it might just as well be sticking into a piece of wood" There can scarcely be any lower rating than this of a person's moral stature.

On this reading of morals, the ultimate moral inadequacy consists in a lack of feeling that is the root of all selfishness. The imperative is implied: "In all interpersonal situations put yourself into the skin of the other, and see if you can contemplate the consequences of your proposed action with equanimity." If we call this frame of mind "sympathetic impartiality," we can elicit from the maxim the view that sympathetic impartiality is the first principle of all morals. This principle is also the logical basis of the golden rule, or the obverse of it, which is frequently heard in Akan ethical talk, namely, "Do not do onto others what you would not that they do onto you." (*Nea wo yonko de ye wo erenye wo de no mfa nye no.*) More literally: What you would not find acceptable if it were done to you by another, do not do to anyone. To be sure, this does not sound, even in our vernacular, as epigrammatic as the normal run of Akan apothegms; still, it provides a solid foundation for the definition of moral worth in its most edifying sense.

COMMUNAL BELONGING

The foregoing account of the Akan perspective on moral first principles, however sketchy, forms the basis of our next question. "In what basic ways do the Akan endeavor to translate their ethical understanding into practical fact?" In this regard the single most important consideration concerns the depth of the Akan sense of the sociality of human existence. Morality is, of course, necessarily social. Thus, any group of humans that have any sense of morals at all—surely, a most minimal species credential—will have some sense of human sociality. But in the moral consciousness of humankind a finely graduated continuum of the intensity of this feeling exists, and it ranges, in an ascending order, from the austerely delimited social sympathies of rigorous individualism to the pervasive commitment and social involvement characteristic of communalism. A commonplace of anthropological wisdom is that African social organization manifests communalism. Akan society is eminently true to this typology.

What this means, more amply, is that Akan society attaches the greatest value to communal belonging. And the way in which a sense of communal belonging is fostered in the individual is through the concentrated stress on kinship identity already foreshadowed in our earlier allusions to the Akan concept of a person. Not only is there what might perhaps be called an ontological basis for this identity in terms of the constituents of personhood, but there is also a distinct normative layer of profound social significance in the concept. Thus conceived, a human person is essentially the center of a thick set of concentric circles of obligations and responsibilities matched by rights and privileges revolving around levels of relationships irradiating from the consanguinity of household kith and kin through the "blood" ties of lineage and clan to the wider circumference of the one human family based on the common possession of the divine spark.

In consequence of this social characteristic in the Akan concept of person, habitual default in duties and responsibilities leads to diminution of one's status as a person in the eyes of the community. Not, of course, that becoming less a person implies that one is unworthy of human rights. On the contrary, a strong sense of the irreducibility of human dignity prevails in Akan thought. However socially benighted or befuddled an individual may be, he or she still remains a direct gift from God incarnated through the intimacy of man and woman. One always remains, in other words, a human being, and as such, deserves basic respect and sympathy. Indeed, as soon as a confirmed social futility begins to look pathologically chronic, animadversion quickly turns into solicitude, and any previous efforts in hortatory correction or in the application of concrete sanctions are redirected toward rehabilitation, usually with the aid of indigenous specialists in bodily and mental health.

Nevertheless, all Akans steeped in the culture or sensitive to surrounding social norms constantly watch and pray lest they be overtaken by the specter of loss of personhood (in any degree). More positively and more optimistically, every cultivated Akan (*Okaniba*) views life as a continual striving after personhood in ever increasing dimensions. The details of this life mission, so to speak, are also the details of the Akan vision of the ethical life.

What, then, in its social bearings, is the Akan ideal of personhood? It is the concept of an individual who through mature reflection and steady motivation is able to carve out a reasonably ample livelihood for self, "family," and a potentially wide group of kin-dependents while also making substantial contributions to the well-being of the larger society. The communalistic orientation of the society means that an individual's images depend rather crucially on the extent to which actions benefit others rather than self, not of course by accident or coincidence but by design. The implied counsel is not, however, one of unrelieved self-denial. Akans are well aware that charity farther afield must start at home. Or, more pertinently, they are apt to point out that one cannot blow a horn on an empty stomach. (*Yede ayaase na ehyen aben.*) Nevertheless, an individual who remains content with self-regarding successes will be viewed as being so circumscribed in outlook as not to merit the title of a real person.

Opportunities for other-regarding exertions in Akan society were and are legion. By the very nature of the traditional economy, which was predominantly agricultural and based on individual self-employment, public works had, as a rule, to be done by voluntary communal labor. Habitual absences, malingering, or half-hearted participation marked one as a useless person (*onipa hunu*) or, by an easily deduced Akan equation, a nonperson (*onye onipa*). In contemporary Ghana (and Ivory Coast), where the Akans live, many public works are financed by mandatory taxes and carried out by professionals with hired labor. Yet, in the villages and small towns especially, a significant portion of such work is still done by voluntary communal labor and voluntary contributions of money and materials.

We face, however, a contemporary complication: with the growth of commerce and industry, including the industry of modern politics, a number of Akans have become very rich and are, in the Akan manner, making voluntary contributions of unprecedented magnitudes to their communities. Their communities, of course, reciprocate in fine eulogistic style and lionize them in other ways as is traditional. So far so good, except for the following circumstance. Some of these people have come by their assets, part of which they so generously donate to the public, through short cuts and other debatable techniques of acquisition. The unfortunate effects that this situation has on the ideals of the young constitute one of the more intractable problems generated by the effect of industrialization on the Akan traditional ethic.

Another aspect of Akan culture flowing from its communalistic outlook that is imperiled by modern conditions—in this case, through atrophy rather than adulteration—is the practice of neighborhood mutual aid. This practice had a deep foundation in Akan values. I have already quoted the Akan adage, *Onipa na ohvia* that affirms through the semantic fecundity of the word *hyia*, both that human interest is the basis of all value and that human fellowship is the most important of human needs. The concepts of *hyia* in the context of the adage are, in fact, a veritable mine of ethical meanings, and bears the seeds of another fundamental thought in the Akan philosophy of life, which is explicit in the maxim *Onipa hyia moa*, meaning that "a human being needs help." The intent of this maxim, however, is not merely to observe a fact, but also to prescribe a line of conduct. The imperative is carried by the word *hyia*, which in this context connotes entitlement: A human being deserves or ought to be helped.

This imperative is born of an acute sense of an essential dependency in the human condition. Dependency is, therefore, also a component of the Akan concept of a person. "A human being" says a noted Akan proverb, "is not a palm tree so as to be self-sufficient" (*Onipa nye abe na ne ho ahyia ne ho*). Indeed, at birth, a human being is not only not self-sufficient but also radically self-insufficient. The human person is totally dependent on others. In due course, through growth and acculturation, acquired skills and abilities reduce this dependency, but it can never be completely eliminated. What, in human affairs, is called self-reliance, is, of course, understood and recommended by the Akans, but its very possibility is predicated on the residue of human dependency. Human beings, therefore, at all times, in one way or another, directly or indirectly, need the help of their kind.

One very standard situation in Akan life that may serve as an illustration of this truth occurred in traditional agriculture, which was generally based on small holdings worked by individual farmers and their households. In such a mode of production it was possible to foresee recurrent stages at which the resources of any one farmer would be insufficient to accomplish a necessary task, for example, the initial clearing of the ground, or the harvesting of cocoa beans from great heaps of pods. In such moments the farmer simply sent word to neighbors that help was needed. Very much as the day follows the night, the people would assemble and with their own implements work together to get the job done speedily and with festive enthusiasm, in full and warranted conviction that when their turn came the gesture would be returned in exactly the same spirit. Anybody who availed himself of the benefits of the system but dragged his feet when the call came from others was liable to be convicted at the bar of public opinion of such fathomless degeneracy as to be branded a social outcast. This type of mutual aid probably occurs in varying intensities in rural communities all over the world; but in traditional Akan society it was so much a part of experience that the Akans actually came to think of life (*obra*) as one continuous drama of mutual aid (*nnoboa*).

In recent times, however, amid the exigencies of urbanization and the increasing, if not yet preponderant, commercialization of agriculture, the ideology of mutual aid is losing hold, and the spirit of neighborhood solidarity, though by no means extinguished, is finding fewer avenues of expression. It has not escaped some leaders of opinion that the traditional ethos of mutual aid might profitably be channelled into a strong movement of modern cooperatives, but so

far organized effort in this direction lacks momentum and its results
are paltry.

PRACTICAL AND CONTEMPORARY MATTERS

Nevertheless, the sense of human solidarity continues to manifest itself quite pervasively in the daily life of the Akans and other peoples
of Ghana for whom these moral characterizations are, in fact, true, if
not to the letter, then at least to the syllable. Happily too, the threat of
individualism posed by urbanization has not yet proved unduly dele-
terious to this national trait. Thus even now a Ghanaian on the coun-
tryside or in a large city, coming on another human being, Ghanaian
or foreigner, in some difficulty, will go out of the way to help. As far
as Ghanaians are concerned, the bad person is one who would walk
away from another on the excuse of some pressing business. Of
course, if "urbani" and other apparent concomitants of moderniza-
tion are not controlled with conscious and rational planning based on
the humane sensitivities of the communalistic ethic, then this fund of
automatic human goodness will bankrupt, and African life will begin
increasingly to experience the Hobbesian rigors of a single-minded
commercialism. The allusion to foreigners prompts a further observation. The sense of human solidarity that we have been discussing
works particularly to the advantage of foreigners, who, in the deeply
felt opinion of the Akans, are doubly deserving of sympathy: first, by
reason of their common humanity; second, by reason of their vulnerability as individuals cut off for the time being from the emotional and
material supports of their kinship environment. Accordingly, when
some time ago an Akan musician and lyricist sang, "*Akwantu mu sem,
Akwantufo ye mmobo,*" (Considering the troubles that can beset a traveler, the plight of a traveler is truly touching), he struck a sympathetic
cord at the depths of the Akan consciousness. Gratified visitors to
Ghana have often been quick to acknowledge the benefits of this
regard.

The allusion to the notion of kinship support reminds us that kinship is the highest value in the Akan community. It is, after all, the
basis of the sense of belonging that gives psychological stability to
each individual (which, incidentally, is why a traveler's absence from
kin strikes the Akans as such hardship). It is also, conversely, the
basis of the obligations in terms of which one's moral standing is as-
sessed.

The smallest and the most intimate Akan kinship unit is the matrilineal household. This includes a person's mother and her mother's

children, his mother's sisters and brothers, the children of the mother's sisters and, at the top, the grandmother. The English words "aunt" and "cousin" fail to capture the depth of kinship feelings corresponding to the relations of mother's sister and mother's sister's children respectively, in spite of their mechanical correctness as translations. In the Akan language the words for mother and mother's children are the same as for mother's sisters and mother's sister's children. Since these relationships already constitute a sizable community then, especially if the grandmother's fertility is at least average, an Akan child will begin life with quite a large sense of belonging and broad, sympathetic support.

The next extension of the circle of kinship relations brings us to the level of the lineage. Here the basic unit consists of a person's grandmother, her children and grandchildren together with the grandmother's brothers and sisters, and the children and grandchildren of her sisters. This unit quickly swells with the culturally legitimate addition of the grandmother's maternal cousins and their descendants. From the point of view of a person's civic existence, this is the most significant circle of relations because, in traditional times, it was through the head of the lineage that a person had political representation.

The lineage, as can easily be imagined, is a quite considerable group of people, but it is small in comparison with the maximal limit of kinship grouping, which is the set of all the people descending from one woman, the clan. For a quick idea of its magnitude, consider that the Akans, now numbering about seven million, trace their collective ancestry to seven women. Clearly individual Akans will never know all their relatives, but they know that they have a million of them.

For practical purposes, however, the household and lineage circles of relations have the most significance in terms of informal rights and obligations. Two illustrations must suffice here. Individual adult members of the lineages may be called on to make financial contributions to rescue one of the fold fallen on hard times, such as freedom-threatening insolvency. By virtue of the powers of arithmetic, this obligation may not necessarily take a heavy toll on individual pocket books. Moreover, reflective individuals will know that they might conceivably have been the beneficiaries.

The next illustration involves a lugubrious subject matter. Bereavement is one of the severest trials of the human psyche. Unfortunately it is recurrent. By both precept and practice Akan traditional culture engages itself, pre-eminently, one might even say, with finding ways to soothe lacerated emotions in such crises. The lineage system incorporates just such a mechanism. In full operation everyone in the lineage is expected to play his part by word, song, dance, and material resource. Nor does the culture leave this to the lineage alone. Friends, neighbors and even indirect acquaintances can always be counted on to help to lighten the burden of sorrows. The framework for this support is the quite elaborate system of the Akan funeral. Despite the excesses created by the rising tide of commercialism and egotistical exhibitionism, the Akan funeral remains an expression of human solidarity at its most heartfelt depth. Proper participation therein is, in Akan eyes, contributory proof of real personhood.

It is clear that socialization in the broad context of the lineage is a school for morality in the Akan culture. Through the kinship channels of the lineage the Akan sense of the social nature of human beings finds its natural expression. Moral life in the wider community is only an extension of a pattern of conduct developed at the lineage level. The fundamental values, some of which we have already outlined, are the same on the two planes, and may be briefly, summarized. A communalistic orientation will naturally prize social harmony. A characteristic Akan, and, as it seems, African way of pursuing this ideal is through decision making by consensus rather than majority opinion. In politics—traditional African politics, not the modern travesties rampant on the continent—this characteristic pursuit leads to a form of democracy very different from the Western variety.

A thoroughgoing consensual approach to social issues can be expected to lead to correspondingly consensual procedures in other areas of social life. A particularly interesting case relates to the Akan reaction to wrongdoing. Though the retributive spirit is not totally absent from reactions, especially at the state level, the predominant tendency to some forms of wrongdoing is to seek compensation or reconciliation or, in cases where extrahuman forces are thought to be estranged, purification. I abstain advisedly from using the word "punishment" in this context; it may well be that there is no unproblematic rendering of this notion in the Akan conceptual framework. The scope of this essay, however, limits our pursuit of this question.

A well-known feature of Akan morals is respect for age. This is intelligible not only from the fact that we are dealing with a society strongly based on kinship relations, which are naturally patterned into hierarchies based on age, but also because in traditional societies, age is associated with knowledge, experience, and wisdom.

Akan moral thinking about sex and marriage also deserves special mention. Here the humanistic and the communalistic aspects of the Akan outlook come into play with interesting results. Because only empirical considerations bearing on human interests are admitted in moral evaluation, such unconditional proscriptions of premarital sex as those found in Christian teaching are absent from the moral rules of the Akan. From the Akan point of view, it is irrational to stop a prospective couple from seeking full knowledge of each other, whether morally, psychologically, or sexually—though, there is, of course, no sexual free-for-all. Still, a nonfurtive relationship between an unmarried man and an unmarried woman need not be restricted to hugging. The only proviso is that the relationship should be aboveboard.

On the other hand, the high value placed on reproductive fertility in a communalistic society based on single-family agriculture will predictably lead to the greatest emphasis being placed on the desirability of marriage and procreation. So much is this the case, that being married with children well raised is part of the necessary condition for personhood in the normative sense. Nonmarrying, nonprocreative persons, however normal otherwise—not to speak of a Casanova equivalent—can permanently forget any prospect of this type of recognition in traditional Akan society.

To understand these facts about the Akan conception of morals does not necessarily mean that we will understand the culture in its entirety, but it does provides us with a sure sense of its foundations.

ROBERT M. VEATCH:

Response to Kwasi Wiredu

I come as a student of comparative ethics to offer a commentary on
the paper of Professor Wiredu. I wish, however, to begin by affirming
the importance of the project before us. Anyone who has taught, as I
have, a course involving cross-cultural comparative medical ethics,
must recognize the tremendous need for serious scholarly accounts of
African and African-American biomedical ethical positions. In my
case, I have simply had to acknowledge to students that there ought
to be a section of the course on these perspectives (and on Latin-
American perspectives), but I have had to plead that neither my
knowledge nor the available literature permitted adequate study of
them.

My practical, clinical goal is to help facilitate good relations
between clinical care-givers and patients. My hypothesis is that if
professional care-givers and patients come to a relation with commitments to different ethical traditions, they will have great difficulty
understanding one another. Specifically, clinicians ought to be able to
know what is medically appropriate for their patients even if their patients' concepts of what is medically right and good are defined by a
system of beliefs and values different from the clinicians. Thus, the
work that is undertaken by this conference and by Professor Wiredu
in particular seems to me of critical importance.

Having affirmed the importance of Professor Wiredu's project, let
me address a few questions to him and to others who are undertaking
the project of this conference.

IS THERE A SINGLE MORAL FOUNDATION OF
AFRICAN CULTURE?

Professor Wiredu provides us with a fascinating account, which he
acknowledges is based on his native knowledge of the Akans of
Ghana. One who is totally an outsider listening to an account of a
tribal or ethnic group is always left with a question of whether there
could be other, equally competent, yet different accounts. I raise this
question only because I know how varied accounts can be of the ethical system of groups with which I am familiar, such as white middle-
class Americans.

I was quite surprised, for example, to learn that African moral
concepts have a generally humanistic orientation, and that morality is
independent from religions in the Akan world view. I am surprised,
in part, because my exposure to the ethical system of the Yoruba in
Nigeria led me to expect the opposite. Given that accounts of white
middle-class American ethics vary, from the very secular and philosophical to the deeply religious, I cannot tell for sure what to make of
Professor Wiredu's description. Is he telling us that all Akans would
concur that their ethical system is humanistic or secular? If so, what,
if anything, can we say about something as complex as "African culture"?

My single most important "teacher" of Yoruba culture was Bolaji
Idowu, a lecturer in Religious Studies at the University of Ibadan.[1]
Based on his work, other Yoruba sources, and my own observations
during two years in Nigeria, my impression is that Yoruba ethics is
intrinsically bound up with religion. As Idowu puts it, "With the
Yoruba, morality is certainly the fruit of religion. They do not attempt
to separate the two."[2] My even sparser sources focusing on East
Africa suggest the same. Godfrey Wilson's essay on "An African
Morality," which is actually an account of the Nyakyusa in what is
now southern Tanzania, treats morality as "right custom sanctioned
by religion."[3] He makes clear that, in his view of the Nyakyusa,
morality, witchcraft, magic, and religion are as intimately connected
as they are in the various anthropological accounts of other African
societies.

Is there a dramatic difference from one African society to another
so that morality for the Akan is radically different in its foundations
from the morality of the Yoruba and the Nyakyusa? If so, that fact
will have important implications for a project that seeks an account of
some general African or African-American morality. Or is it possible
that different analysts will give different accounts of Akan, Yoruba,
and Nyakyusa moral foundations? This question may be critical to

the link between religions and the grounding of morality in African-American culture.

SUBSTANTIVE NORMATIVE ETHICS

I turn now to substantive issues in normative ethics. I was struck by the fact that Professor Wiredu's account does not easily translate into the standard language of an Anglo-American analytical description of a normative ethic. I attempted a thought experiment to convert the account into the language with which I am most accustomed. I want to raise a few questions.

Is this a legitimate enterprise, however, or would Professor Wiredu say that any such translation, in principle, corrupts the ethic from the other culture? Would a proponent of an African ethic argue as, for example, American feminists might, that any attempt to convert their ethic into the standard ethic of virtues, principles, and axiology destroys it?

Recognizing that I am purposely inviting such criticism, let me provide my normative account as a translation of Professor Wiredu's description of Akan ethics. First, it seems that the Akan ethics described by Professor Wiredu is decidedly consequentialistic. According to him, for the Akan, "What is good in general is what promotes human interests." Then, there is apparently a clear altruistic dimension, as seen in the Akan version of the Golden Rule that Professor Wiredu cited. To what extent, therefore, do Akan ethics reduce to a kind of utilitarianism—including its support of paternalism (as in the Golden Rule) and its theoretical indifference to distributive matters?

I raise the question not only because the appeal to human interests has a utilitarian ring, but because I find in Professor Wiredu's account the absence of other major principles that would surface in a mainstream Anglo-American ethical theory. First, it seems to me that such a utilitarian ethic would be in conflict with a Hippocratic medical ethic focusing on the welfare of the individual patient. Second, I see no reference in it to autonomy, justice, or the other standard principles of veracity; or to promise-keeping, privacy, or a prohibition on killing.

My own modest knowledge of the literature on African ethical systems supports the inference that these principles do not play a central role in other African ethical systems either, a conclusion also supported by my relatively brief experience with the Yoruba. My interactions with school teachers, students, university faculty, and medical professionals in Nigeria yielded little evidence of the ethical principles that are at the heart of Western liberal political philosophy, especially in its American manifestation. Two examples will have to suffice.

First, in the local hospitals in the community of Ogbomosho, my American liberalism and sensitivity immediately rebelled when I saw patients treated without any semblance of respect for privacy, right to self-determination, or equality. Patients were cared for in very public areas and were subject to examinations in circumstances that would have generated charges of gross violations of privacy in the United States. I could easily overhear patient-physician encounters that caused embarrassment to my provincial American sense of confidentiality. When my wife or I sought medical care from the clinic, as relatively high-status whites, we were routinely escorted to the front of the line. This caused us not only embarrassment but also outrage; we protested until we were informed that our resistance had been interpreted as lack of appreciation for their hospitality. It was clear that neither privacy nor American egalitarianism prevailed.

My second example involves the regimen at the local school in which my wife and I taught. There the British system of hazing young students by designating them as virtual servants of fifth formers clashed with our American egalitarianism. When we instinctively sided with the younger ones, we created chaos among the students and teachers. Moreover, since I was trained in neuro-pharmacology, I bore the closest resemblance to a health officer available in the school. I was officially the head of the dispensary. In this role as well I encountered two problems. I began to realize that my concepts of what counted as a medical problem differed dramatically from those of my African students. I worried about malaria; they worried about something called "general weakness of the body." I maintained my well-ingrained medical conservatism, being extremely cautious about dispensing drugs like codeine; they, on the other hand, were eager to use medications in ways I thought useless or terribly dangerous. Most striking to me, however, was that everyone, including the Africans, expected me to impose my judgments on the students. I ended up paternalistically wanting to impose antipaternalism on them.

I was left with the nagging question that I would raise for Professor Wiredu: Was there a sense of autonomy and justice there that I could not see, or was their ethic grounded in other commitments? Or are Western concepts of autonomy and justice alien concepts? My impression is that the Ibo of Eastern Nigeria have a different sense of authority and status differentials than do Westerners in general.

IMPLICATIONS FOR AFRICAN-AMERICAN BIOETHICS

I have one last question that I want to address to the conference participants as much as to Professor Wiredu. It is one of the key questions of this conference. What are the implications for an *African-American* biomedical ethics?

It seems like an account of African-American ethics might plausibly find its roots in Africa. But if there are many African cultures and many accounts of those cultures, will we be able to trace the connecting links? Moreover, even a cursory familiarity with African-American ethics impresses one with its emphasis on its religious grounding. Normatively, one is impressed with its emphasis on autonomy and equality, freedom and justice. For obvious reasons, from the emergence of an ethic of emancipation to the recent days of civil rights, African-American ethics has taught us a great deal about the principles of liberty and justice. Where did they come from? What are their links to Africa?

Is there something inherently wrong with trying to describe African-American bioethics using these Anglo categories? Is it, for example, a vestige of liberalism (when communitarianism would be more appropriate) to suggest that accounts of African-American bioethics would have more in common with feminist and Marxist theory than with Anglo-analytical philosophy? I hope that papers such as Professor Wiredu's will help us begin to shed light on these problems. Patients and providers who stand in the African-American tradition need to know. Those interacting with them need to know as well.

NOTES

1. Bolagi, Idowu, *Olodumare—God in Yoruba Belief* (London: Longmans, Green and Co. Ltd., 1962), 144-168.
2. Ibid., 146.
3. Godfrey, Wilson, "An African Morality", *Cultures and Societies of Africa*, ed. Simon and Phoebe Ottenberg (New York: Random House; 1960), 345-365.

Response to Kwasi Wiredu

My commentary will incorporate my response to Professor Wiredu's paper and some thoughts stimulated by other contributions to this forum. I am impressed by the analytic focus on language, meaning, and the definitions of terms. I wonder, however, if these traditionally accepted methods of intellectual inquiry of European-American civilization may not in and of themselves inhibit or restrict an appropriate analysis of African-American moral foundations. In a variety of ways, we have asked ourselves that question. As part of a scholarly endeavor we must seek a common framework and operational definitions with which we can agree and work. For me, the problem of who defines the terms and whence comes the language is central. Clearly what is viewed as authentic in this society is of European origin. If we accept this reality, and I believe we must, then the real challenge facing us is the appropriateness of our framework for understanding an African world view.

Our examination of the moral foundations and the obligations and duties that emanate from those foundations raises questions about whether knowledge of Africa in any way informs our understandings of African-American thought. What continuities do we see? Can we attribute any similarities to the African heritage? What other explanations and interpretations are there? How can we test and validate our assumptions in a more "scientific" and "rational" manner, or is that in fact necessary, in light of the concerns that such a focus is not an African or African-American way of knowing?

The inquiry at this conference provides an expansion of our knowledge base and provides important linkages to what we are calling European-American or Eurocentric concepts with African-American or Afrocentric concepts. From a clinician's perspective, the inquiry raises the possibility of finding answers that might improve patient care. If there are insights and information about African-Americans that are different from the insights and information with which the culture generally operates, then their discovery has implications for care and caregivers. We are, in fact, examining the efficacy of a new framework for clinical care. If our investigations should determine that African-Americans differ from others in terms of values, morals, and world views, such knowledge may warrant new or different responses to such issues as life-sustaining treatment, self-determination, autopsy requests, organ donation and transplantation, and reproductive technologies. Finally, this inquiry has significant implications for public policy formation; as we become cognizant of differences, we must also accommodate differences so that appropriate policies may be implemented.

As I focus specifically on Dr. Wiredu's presentation, I have some questions about his statements on religious traditions. Perhaps with further elucidation, we can obtain a better understanding. I find in Dr. Wiredu's comments too narrow a definition of religion and perhaps a slight contradiction. Professor Wiredu speaks of African religion as purely intellectual, yet he later mentions that a person comes directly from God and contains a speck of divine substance. I do not read or interpret this latter comment as an intellectual construct. Further discussion is needed to determine the extent to which African traditions and cultures contain more than intellectual religion and are really a unity of religion and human existence. The sense that African-Americans make of the world incorporates this idea, which I believe emanates from African cultures.

Professor Wiredu observes that morality is universal, but that different peoples, groups, and individuals have different understandings of it. Is this a position of ethical relativism? We African-Americans, I believe, tie our notions of morality to the search for meaning in the context of American life. Does our search for meaning and our attempt to create social and moral order differ in fact from that of the dominant group in this country? Do the answers that we find and construct in any way differ? Do the behaviors that result from our understandings in any way differ? Specifically, do our behaviors differ vis-à-vis an understanding of medicine and medical technology? Are there differences in our values or simply in our priorities?

Professor Wiredu's descriptions of African conceptions of morality should be examined for their relevance to African-American culture. He has described a humanistic, person-centered orientation, a moral foundation, a world view, and a communalistic belief system: indeed, a system that holds that human fellowship is the most important human need. This description is in contrast to the Anglo-analytic philosophy that views morality as a cerebral and introspective enterprise. That does not appear to be the African way.

Although there may be some independence of morality from religion in Africa, the good is defined as that which promotes human interests; it is person-centered. The good is utilitarian and practical, but it is driven by a person-centered focus. And it includes unconditional reverence and absolute trust in a Supreme Being. Morality is an individual responsibility; a familial and social responsibility to others; and, lastly, a community responsibility which in practical fact and action touches on justice. African traditions dislike injustice. Not only is the correctness of conduct tied up with passion, but moral inadequacy consists in a lack of feeling that is the root of all selfishness. Wiredu states that a strong sense of the irreducibility of human dignity, basic respect, and sympathy for others undergirds and drives the moral foundation of African peoples.

Conceptually, personhood conveys concomitant personal and social responsibilities. It is not enough just to be or to think abstractly. Rather, as Wiredu indicates, through mature reflection and steady motivation, one should be able to do; one should be able to get things done and to carve out a reasonably ample livelihood for self, for family, for community. Being is doing. African traditions take a consensual approach to decision making. Recently, I found a wonderful book entitled, "*Trabelin On*" by Mechal Sobel. Sobel attempts to make a connection between African culture and African-American life in terms of the journey from slavery to the Afro-Baptist faith. She tells us that many West African world views did use consensus to coalesce in African-American culture. So, perhaps, West African cultures can be understood in this country as one whole.

Sobel's book is an attempt to reconcile Eurocentric ways of understanding and African ways of knowing. She describes the process of unification, adaptation, and change that took place as slavery moved into this country and as Africans became African-Americans. Many contradictory values were absorbed, resulting in the evolution of the distinctly American Baptist and Methodist churches. Sobel views this evolution as an in-depth reintegration of "the Black soul," and locates it in the creation of the Afro-Baptist faith. She describes a new "sacred cosmos" and a moral foundation that integrates African and Baptist elements into a unified whole.

John Mbiti, another African scholar, notes the difficulty that having so few written documents makes to the study of the religions and philosophies of African peoples. Important elements are not on paper, but in people's hearts, minds, oral history, rituals, and religious personages. Perhaps this is the reason that both Mbiti and Sobel speak of belief and action as one, as belonging to a single whole in African culture.[1] Conduct, not thought, is of value and is meant to be judged. Immorality is anything that hinders the development of the community. Here again, the world view is humanistic; it is one that believes in "being"—being with intelligence, being tied concomitantly to time and place, being shared in spirit.[2] In many ways, African-American culture is an amalgam of these concepts.

Several problems continue to surface as we proceed to describe and attempt to document the above observations. We must be careful not to pick and choose subjectively the characteristics of African-American culture that we think mesh with African-American traditions. The relationship of the social sciences to the work of philosophy is important here. The inquiry demands a multidisciplinary, communalistic, and holistic focus.

African-American social scientists have identified continuities between African and African-American cultures. Billingsley, Hill, and Staples discuss the strong kinship ties, the role flexibility and the communalistic, humanistic orientation of many African-American families.[3] Kochman and Pasteur describe the expressiveness, emotion, passion, and nonformalistic ways of looking at the world to be found among African-Americans.[4] Still needed are further and more in-depth exploration of the ways in which these characteristics, so similar to African characteristics, manifest themselves in African-Americans' behavior and moral reasoning. Are African-Americans more concrete and personal than other Americans in interactions and responses, particularly in biomedical ethics or biomedical encounters? As patients, are we more concrete and personal? Are we more responsive to the concrete and personal than to the abstract? If in fact individual autonomy is valued less than group autonomy, what implications does this fact have for those living in a society that places tremendous emphasis on autonomy?

My own observation is that, conceptually, injustice for African-Americans is more personal than abstract, a notion very visibly and tangibly learned from the African tradition. Injustice is viewed by African-Americans primarily in terms of community. If something is not for the good of the community, not humanistic, not communalistic, it is unjust. Feelings and emotions are a guide, a framework for the moral foundation as opposed to reason, to rational or objective thought. If this observation should hold up under further scrutiny, we must reflect on the significance of the communal consciousness for public policy decisions.

As I view African-Americans in relation to their African heritage, I see a blending of the humanistic and the communalistic. Reasoning and reason are not separate. Reason and spirituality are interrelated; humankind is not purely autonomous, nor should we strive to be. Personhood and justice are intertwined. There is a similarity, I find, between the feminist perspective on justice and that of African-Americans.

A most difficult problem for me has to do with the process and mechanisms by which the mores of a culture are transmitted. Who determines what is valued, replaced, usurped, or altered by other values? We need more rigorous examination of these questions. A multidisciplinary process is clearly required for comprehensive inquiry. What Dr. Wiredu has described and what this conference has addressed is, in fact, a fluid evolving process—continually changing, because the culture, the moral foundations of this society, inclusive of its Euro-and Afrocentric components are changing dramatically.

We ask, "Where are we now?" From whence have we come? Where are we going? Where might we go? And finally, what are the implications for those of us who continue to search for better ways to care for people.

NOTES

1. John S. Mbiti, *African Religions and Philosophy* (New York: Praeger, 1969), 5.

2. Mechal Sobel, *"Trabelin On": The Slave Journey to an Afro-Baptist Faith* (Princeton: Princeton University Press, 1988), 219.

3. Andrew Billingsley, *Black Families in White America* (Englewood Cliffs, New Jersey: Prentice Hall, 1968); Robert Hill, *The Strengths of Black Families* (New York: Emerson Hall Publishers, 1972); Robert Staples, *The Black Family: Essays and Studies* (Belmont, California: Wadsworth Co., 1978).

4. Thomas Kochman, *Black and White Styles in Conflict* (Chicago: University of Chicago Press, 1981); Alfred Pasteur and Ivory Tolson, *Roots of Soul* (New York: Anchor-Doubleday, 1982).

KWASI WIREDU

The African Concept of Personhood

In 1979, President Kaunda of Zambia gave give high praise to then Prime Minister of Britain, Mrs. Margaret Thatcher, for her unexpected constructiveness during the last series of negotiations that led to the termination of white minority rule in Zimbabwe. He said that she was "truly a person," and he immediately provided a key to this choice of words. In Zambian language and culture, personhood is not an automatic quality of the human individual; it is something to be achieved, and the higher the achievement, the higher the credit. On this showing, the "Iron Lady" received very high marks indeed. The semantics of personhood in the language of the Zambians is similar to the semantics of personhood accepted by the Akans of Ghana and the Ivory Coast.

The word for person in Akan is *onipa*. It will be understood at once that the word harbors an ambiguity. In one sense *onipa* designates "a human being"; in another sense, it designates an individual who has attained a commendable status in society. The ambiguity is quite benign, however, for the meaning is always clearly determined by its context.

There is here a remarkable contrast of languages. In English, "person" does not suggest an attribution susceptible of degrees; an entity is or is not a person. True, in English we may call someone "personable," which is a descriptive remark; but that can scarcely be said to reveal a new sense of the word "person." This is why President Kaunda had to explain his wording. In contrast to English, the language of the Akans and many African peoples construes personhood as an ideal that may or may not be realized and to which one may approximate in varying degrees.[1] What accounts for this duality of meaning?

Why does this word that so many African languages use for what the English call a "person" have a normative layer of meaning? The answer, I suggest, lies in the deeply communalistic notion of human existence entertained among the peoples of Africa. A person is, one might say, analytically social. Aristotle says that man is by nature political. If "political" is interpreted to presuppose government, this is false; in traditional times some ethnic groups in Africa had no government.[2] A human being is social before he or she is political; in African thinking, the necessary sociality of the human status is primarily of the kinship type, which, of all human relations, is the most natural. And since society presupposes some rules of harmony defining a system of values, the normative bent of the concept of a person in the African context is clearly inevitable.

There are two levels of normative significance in the African concept of person. In the first, personhood is a status conditional on certain social achievements; in the second a descriptive component is added to the concept. We will come to the latter component and its normative implications in due course. But let me comment first on the level of normative meaning, which was unavoidably touched on in my discussion of "The Moral Foundations of African Culture."

ACHIEVING PERSONHOOD

The first prerequisite of personhood is marriage and procreation, obvious dictates of a communalistic ethic. It follows by a rather immediate inference, that an infant is not yet a person. But any fears that this notion is a cultural license for child abuse should be laid to rest by our recollection that the Akan beings called *onipa* are never less than human beings, or beings developmentally achieving human being. Obviously, an *onipa* is never less than a human being, and any progeny of human parentage is an *onipa*. Akans hold that there is a divine element in the nature of all human beings. On this ground alone, everyone, young or old, is entitled to a minimum of respect and dignity and a full complement of human rights.[3] Moreover, because of their relative helplessness, infants are viewed as needing greater love and care than adults. At the same time, they are viewed as more wonderful than adults, for in them are lodged more or less limitless, undissipated potentialities.

In the case of adults, there is usually not much to tease or intrigue the mind about the magnitude or direction of their potentialities; they have had time to give indications of them and to develop or dissipate them, as the case may be. But an infant is a center of virtually untouched possibilities, and there is no knowing how it may shape the world. A certain sense of wonderment prevails. From time to time, a child prodigy will burst forth to the attention of adults. Then the direction of its abilities will be known but not their outcomes. Moreover, the very precociousness of the phenomenon induces a mystified curiosity. An Akan adult will use the phrase *adwadaa nyame* in reference to the child in question. Literally, the phrase means "child as God," revealing a certain degree of awe. Quite often, especially in lyrics, the phrase is used more abstractly to express a generalized sense of mystified wonderment somewhat in the spirit of Wordsworth's "The child is the father of the man."

At the death of an infant, no funeral ceremonies are permitted in Akan society. Indeed, if the deceased is a baby, the parents are encouraged to eat normally and pursue all the occupations of more cheerful times. The reason for this is common sense, though it is sometimes given a "spiritual" slant. If grief and depression, which are understood to be quite natural in such circumstances, are not quickly counteracted, thoughts of replacing the loss and the acts necessary thereto may be unduly delayed. From the Akan point of view, the death of an infant is an unnatural termination of life that cries for generic restoration.

A more irreducibly cosmological reason, additional to the foregoing, is that a funeral is, in part, a formalized send-off for the departing "soul" on the journey to the world of our ancestors.[4] But an infant soul, not having reached personhood, cannot become an ancestor, and does not, therefore, have a ticket for that journey. A theory of selective reincarnation postulates a second chance in the world of mortals, for the completion of a full term of life. Therefore, however interpreted, the absence of funerals on the demise of infants concerns the prolongation of their lives rather than lack of respect for their status.

On proper consideration, then, the Akan custom in question can be seen to be far removed from any cultural predilection for child abuse. In all likelihood, wickedness is, in terms of overall statistics, evenly distributed among the different peoples of the world; but the particular manifestation of wickedness that is seen in child abuse is, in fact, rare in Akan culture. Speaking personally, I was perhaps aware of some child abuse in the Akan culture in the form of the occasional excess of draconian spanking, but I had to come to the United States in middle age to discover the multifarious varieties of child victimization.

It is instructive, furthermore, to note the differing ways in which an infant and a non-achieving adult are considered to fall short of personhood. The infant is not a person because it is still in preparation for that status. Adult "do-littles," on the other hand, fail to be persons for lack of pulling their weight. Opprobrium attaches to the second condition of life; none to the first.

There are, of course, many ways in which an individual can be seen as not pulling his weight. It is obvious, for example, from the first condition of personhood that a life of confirmed celibacy will be seen in this light. From a traditional Akan point of view, only an inveterate waywardness can account for a lifestyle so prejudicial to the perpetuation of the lineage, the ethnic group, or, on a larger view, the species, unless it be due to impotence. The latter incapacity would typically elicit profuse sympathy from relatives and other well-wishers, and no lack of help, including encouragement to widen the scope of partners and the provision, if necessary, of facilities for physical and psychiatric treatment. It will be perceived as a matter of the gravest import, for, unless the problem can be overcome, personhood will remain elusive, even if the attitude of the public is more of pity than contempt.[5]

Other ways of failing to achieve personhood suggest conditions helpful for attaining that standing. It is not enough just to marry and have children; the household should be amply provided for and wisely administered, jointly, of course, between both spouses. More than this, one is expected to make concrete material contributions to the well-being of one's lineage, which is quite a sizable group of people. A series of events in the lineage, such as marriages, births, illnesses and deaths, will give rise to urgent obligations. The individual who is able to meet these in a timely and adequate manner is the true person. There are more tests for personhood connected with lineage levels of existence, but the above suffice as general examples.

It must be conceded that the conditions of personhood are, indeed, quite exacting. But it is to be observed that they are also correlated with rights and privileges, which, in times of trial and tribulation, can make all the difference between success and failure.

So far, our considerations in regard to the normative requirements for personhood have revolved around duties which, broadly speaking, may be termed "self-regarding." In a communalistically shaped consciousness, household and lineage must be inextricably bound up with the conception of the ego and its own needs. But there are "other-regarding" criteria of personhood of community-wide scope that are no less crucial. Where public projects can only be accomplished by means of voluntary communal labor, full participation is, naturally expected of any individual who claims title as a respectable member of society, which every person is conceived to be.[6] Individuals worthy of the title must bear their fair share of the burden of defending their community, which in traditional times fell to an inclusive citizens' army. Human beings must also take part, as appropriate, in the proper governance of their community and in activities designated to achieve therein a harmony of interests, good will, and the flourishing of people in work, relaxation, and the taming of grief.

FREEDOM AND RESPONSIBILITY

The desiderata of personhood recounted here, pretty much exhaust, in a summary way, the normative connotation of the concept and presuppose, when taken together, the ability to act on the basis of rational reflection. They presuppose also, in the normal run of things, a sound body and a reasonably strong and consistent motivation seasoned with a good dose of human sympathy. Leaving the physical qualifications aside for the time being, it may be noted that these mental attributes play a philosophically instructive role in Akan evaluations of human action. An adult of irrational and erratic habits will bring on her or himself the judgment "so and so is not a person" (*onye onipa*). Nevertheless, such a one will not necessarily fall outside the pale of rational persuasion or moral correction. Indeed, the utterance of the judgments in the hearing of the subject will, in itself, be an exercise in moral persuasion.

Household and lineage personages can be expected to accentuate that note and press earnestly for character reform; for, apart from anything else, in the communalistic milieu of Akan society, disgrace for one member of the lineage is, to some extent, disgrace for all. In many cases these efforts will bear fruit and the individual concerned will be urged to reappraise and redirect his or her line of conduct. Indeed, one of the most agonizing moments in the life of an Akan is being constrained in this situation to ask, "Am I ever going to become a person?" (*Se me be ye nipa ni?*) This is a supreme moment of self-questioning that can, in some cases, have a transforming effect.

But suppose that in spite of the combined efforts of mentors and negative critics, an individual continues unalterably in the path of moral error or irrational idiosyncrasy. Akan observers will then conclude that moral deterioration has passed into psychological pathology; they will discontinue moral criticism and look for medical and psychiatric treatment for the individual. (Often they may suspect the malevolent intervention of some extrahuman forces.) At this stage the individual is no longer deemed responsible. *Enye onoa*, it is said; literally, "It is not he," or *enye nania*, "It is not his eyes." The interpretation of both these sayings is that the person is not himself, that is, not responsible for his behavior.

Here now is the philosophical point. In Akan speech the saying cited above corresponds to what in English we would call "the absence of free will." Thus, in Akan, the concept of freedom in metaphysical contexts is the same as the concept of responsibility. Thus, there is not one problem of freedom or free will and a separate problem of responsibility, as there seems to be in the English expression, "the problem of free will *and* responsibility." The problem in Akan is simply, "When is an individual responsible?" And the answer in this brief account of the Akan approach to deviant conduct is that an individual is responsible to the extent that his conduct is can be modified through rational persuasion or moral correction. Conversely, an individual is not responsible to the extent that his behavior cannot be modified through rational persuasion or moral correction. For the equivalence in terms of freedom, substitute "free" for "responsible" and "unfree" for "not responsible."

This position has some very interesting philosophical implications. For example, the question of determinism, namely, whether all events are caused, has no direct bearing on the question of freedom. The relevant question is not whether a given piece of conduct has any causes, but the kind of causes that it has. Whatever the causes, if, on the way to human development, they have led to a pattern of conduct open to modification through rational considerations, the agent concerned is free; otherwise not. The qualification "on the way to human development" is absolutely crucial, for this conception of freedom or responsibility is logically controlled by the ideal of personhood.

A real *onipa* is a living being of human parentage who, through the biological, psychological, cognitive, and moral apprenticeship of a childhood exposed to moral persuasion and correction, has come to develop moral sensibilities and rational habits conducive to a productive and edifying life in society. An apparently human individual who, through a brave-new-world style of acculturation, comes to display the same pattern of behavior as a result of being subjected to selective electrical shocks, would hardly count as a responsible agent, for his manner of development is not the manner of human development.

Akan thought is explicitly deterministic. Among the most popular of our proverbs are the following:

1. Everything has its explanation. (*Biribiara wo ne nkyerease.*)
2. Nothing ever happens for no reason. (*Biribiara nsi kwa.* Literally, "Nothing happens for nothing.")
3. If nothing had touched the dry palm branches, they would not have rattled. (*Se bribi ankoka papa a anka erenye krada.*)
4. If Birebire had not come, there would have been no calamity.[7] (*Birebire amma a amane mma.*)

Yet, there is no hint in Akan thinking that this determinism creates any problem for human responsibility. And rightly so.[8] On this ground, one may be tempted to associate the Akan view with the Western theory of "soft determinism," the theory that free will is compatible with determinism. But there is an important rider in the fact that soft determinism supposes a dual problem of freedom and responsibility. The Akan view, on my interpretation, knows only one problem of responsibility or freedom. The difference may be subtle, but it is very significant.

Other implications of the Akan view are, more briefly, that the question of free will is a normative question, not a descriptive one. Moreover, free will is susceptible of degrees, some individuals being more free than others with respect to a given sphere of conduct, and no one being free to perfection in any regard. To this may be added the further implication that the same individual may be relatively free with respect to one theater of activity and relatively unfree with respect to another. These particulars make the view in question strikingly different from its nearest affiliate in Western philosophy, namely, soft determinism.

But different or not, the question of its truth or falsehood is a separate matter, and the fact that it is drawn from the Akan language and culture provides no clue either way. I happen to think that the Akan view is, in fact, correct. If so, it should, in principle, be arguable with all due elaboration in any language and, in particular, in English. But to do that is not part of my task for this occasion. Suffice it to say, a little more concretely, that some notable theories on the subject in Western philosophy, seem, in some respects, to be oriented in the same direction. Thus Moritz Schlick in his "When Is a Man Responsible?" barely falls short of the realization that there is only one problem of freedom or responsibility.[9] And John Hospers in a much-reprinted pair of papers on the same subject is, in some particulars, of one mind with the Akans, perhaps especially on the definition of responsibility, in spite of apparent "hard" deterministic lapses in some elaborate parts of papers.[10]

From the point of view of our present discussion, the significance of these remarks on the freedom of the will lies in their insight into the complexity of the Akan concept of personhood. To recap the core of the idea, a person is a human individual cognizant of morality and capable of rational self-control and productive living. It follows necessarily that a true person will be possessed to some degree of free will in various domains of human life.

Personhood is open-ended on one side. One can theoretically ascend higher and higher, achieving ever superior levels of personhood with possible gains in free will. But the downward path has a definite bottom line. Past this line, one cannot retain the status of personhood, though one can, provided the descent is not too steep, remain a human being capable of some free choice and residually amenable to rational considerations. An individual at this juncture of existence stands in an uncertain equilibrium. He or she will pull up into the relatively redeeming regions of personhood or sink past another bottom line into "unfreedom," through causes that are largely inscrutable.[11] But even in unfreedom an individual will still remain a human being, possessed of a certain irreducible value.

THE LIFE PRINCIPLE

What, then, is a human being? This question is very relevant to our concerns because, although not all human beings are persons in the normative sense, still, one cannot be a person without being a human being. Moreover, it is the constituents of a person that determine his or her kinship links, which for the Akans are a matter of the greatest importance for the existence of a person. The most critical constituent of a human being is something the Akans call *okra*. This is a speck of God that the Supreme Being offers as a direct gift for the making of a new individual. It is the life principle. Its departure means death and leaves behind only a corpse. In English translation the *okra* is often called the "soul." This translation is extremely problematic, but let us observe here that a human individual is regarded as an embodied *okra*. The body (*nipadua*, literally, "bodily tree") is the organic growth of a biological foundation that is jointly laid by man and woman when they unite in the mating process. In that process the mother contributes the *mogya*, literally, "the blood," and the father contributes *ntoro*, literally, "semen." Both contributions have social significance. The *mogya* is the basis of lineage identity, while the *ntoro* is the basis of membership in a kinship grouping of a mostly ceremonial significance. Around both linkages revolve a set of social obligations, rights, and privileges characteristic of a communalistic existence. Thus the descriptive fact of being the organic outcome of biological input from mother and father is seen to have important normative implications. Equally important is the normative implication of the divine element in the human constitution, which, if it is a fact, is a descriptive one. In virtue of that element, absolutely everyone, regardless of race, gender, or achievement is entitled to a certain degree of respect and consideration. In other words, every human being has a prima facie duty to help any human being in need of help, to eschew acts of gratuitous disrespect, and to give due recognition to his or her human rights. This is the point of the renowned Akan maxim to the effect that "everyone is the child of God, and none the child of the earth." Akans are likely to remind backsliders with the phrase, *Onipa nua ne onipa,* "A human being is the sibling of a human being," that is, all human beings are brothers and sisters.

The normative implications of the Akan concept of personhood should be carefully distinguished from the normative component of the concept itself. In the first half of this discussion, considerable attention was given to the latter component of the meaning of personhood. We now need to address in like manner the descriptive component which, as we will shortly see, entails important ontological clarifications. For example, the doctrine that there is a speck of divine substance in the human being is filled with ontological implications. To these I shall refer in due course. But, first, let us take up, again, the matter of biological constituents.

PHYSICAL CONSTITUENTS AND PERSONAL PRESENCE

Perhaps the most unproblematic constituent of a human being in the Akan concept of personhood is the *mogya,* "the blood principle." The thought of it is closely bound up with the thought of the physical existence of the human individual. Yet, we will find in this particular case, as in other Akan conceptions, that it pays to steer clear of the sharp physical/nonphysical duality that is so often found in Western philosophy. This idea becomes even clearer in connection with the paternal constituent of the human constitution. The *ntoro* is the semen, something biological. But it gives rise, in the human make-up, to something called *sunsum,* that which is responsible for the unique personal presence that each individual has. A person with a commanding personal presence has a strong *sunsum;* a less impressive person has a weak *sunsum.* (The Akan words translated in this context as "strong" and "weak" mean "heavy" and "light," respectively.) A strong *sunsum* is able to resist or repel the attacks of malevolent extrahuman forces, such as witchcraft, while a weak one may be hurt by such forces or even destroyed with consequent illness or death.

If witchcraft and similar alleged phenomena are nonphysical, then they are suggestive of nondualistic continuities in this conceptual framework. This impression is further accentuated when it is noted that the Akans seem traditionally to have believed that in dreams the *sunsum* actually leaves the body and goes out to engage in all the adventures and misadventures that are dreamt of in human slumber. The idea itself is, surely, of questionable coherence, but it suggests very clearly that in the *sunsum* we are dealing with a quasi-physical conception. It is most certainly not conceived as "spiritual" in the Cartesian sense, that is, it is not thought of as being totally extensionless. In its capacity as *dramatis persona*, it is credited with physical exploits, not to speak of mischiefs.[12]

Moreover, the *sunsum* is not ontologically shielded from damage and destruction as spiritual substances of the Cartesian variety are supposed to be. Indeed, according to the account of one of the best authorities on Akan thought, the *sunsum* is "not divine but perishes with the man."[13] This is plausible, first because the *sunsum* is an emanation from a biological source, namely, the father's semen; second, because it is an undeniable fact that traditional Akans believe the *sunsum* to be open to attack and destruction, and third, because, in any case, if the *sunsum* were supposed to survive the death of its human possessor, there would be quite a chaotic ontological situation in the world of the dead. The latter is especially true since the *okra*, considered as a portion of the Supreme Being itself is also thought to be immortal and to become a guardian of the affairs of the clan as an ancestor. Logically, it is not easy to see how the two types of survivors would sort out the inevitable conundrum of identity if they should meet. On the other hand, it is easy to see the wisdom of avoiding the hypothesis that leads to it. Not that the Akans are innocent of all metaphysical solecisms, but it seems needless to attribute that of the immortality of the *sunsum* to them, on the evidence of some of the things that they are known to say about it.

When, therefore, the *sunsum* is rendered into English as "spirit" and is declared to constitute a spiritual dimension of human personality, as is so often done, it is not too alarmist to express fear of an uncritical superimposition of alien categories on Akan thought. At best *sunsum* are spirits only in a non-Cartesian sense in which, for example, the apparitions that are celebrated by Western spiritualists are supposed to be spirits. These are neither fully material nor fully immaterial and that is what is meant by saying that they are quasi-material or quasi-physical. In terms of imagery, these "spirits" are, in fact, remarkably material. They are allegedly seen in human shape or heard as human voices, although supposedly dead. They differ significantly from actual human beings in that they are not supposed to be impeded by locked doors or iron bars. Neither, allegedly, are they restrained by the speed limitations that restrain human motion.

The same is, in principle, true of the *sunsum*. They are not normally perceptible through the senses. But people with trained or treated eyes or ears, for example, are supposed to be able to see or hear *sunsum* entities. Nothing is more common in the extrasensory talk of Akan traditional healers than the claim to see all sorts of such entities around the homes, the street corners, and the fields—places where Akans not endowed with such occult powers walk in serene ignorance.

There is another sense in which the word "spirit" may be used for the *sunsum*. It arises from the following circumstance of usage. As a constituent of a human beings, the *sunsum* is supposed to be something that generates an individual's personal presence. But in a common turn of phrase, the word is often used directly to refer to the personal presence itself. This extension is quite natural. Thinking of an individual's personal presence is not very different from thinking of one's dynamism, charisma, or spiritedness.

It is also quite natural to extend this usage to groups and organizations of people. For example, one may have heard of the *sunsum* of the Ashanti nation in historical times. This was supposed to be enshrined in what was known as the "Golden Stool," the symbol of Ashanti national power. It is conceivable that some have thought of this political soul as an entity actually located in that metal structure, but it is highly unlikely that those who formulated the concept of the national *sunsum* in the stool had such a material understanding.

In 1979, in Ghana, electioneering campaigns leading to the installation of an elected government featured a political party that called itself the party with *sunsum*. It can hardly be supposed that Ghanaians imagined an actual entity at party headquarters, perhaps lodged in a safe, called a *sunsum*. Rather, it was apparently clear that the meaning of *sunsum* in this case was the party dynamism. One might also have expressed the same idea by saying that they were the party of spirit.

The message and its style has an unquestionable cultural appeal, and the party actually won the elections. It would, of course, be simple-minded to suggest that the victory was in the slogan, but one cannot suppose that it was absolutely unconnected with it. Meanwhile, the metaphorical character of the *sunsum* was not lost on a certain flight lieutenant, who, when he decided to seize power from the government of the party with *sunsum* and disband that same party, took up arms, not witchcraft, and made a swift job of it.

Whether or not there is an actual entity in human beings to which the degree of personal presence, dynamism, spirit, or charisma, can be traced, it is clear that the Akans are highly sensitive to the dimension of personality designated by these concepts. I am tempted to use the phrase "the charisma principle" to sum up this aspect of personhood.

Now we return to the *okra*, the life principle in humans and we can be brief in our treatment of it, in view of the foregoing. Much as in the case of the *sunsum*, the *okra* is in fact a quasi-material conception and very different from any Cartesian or neo-Cartesian concept of the soul. The apparent similarity between the two types of concept, namely, that both are joined to a doctrine of immorality, can be quickly unscrambled by noting that the Akan notion of immorality is quasi-material.[14] That the general African world of the dead is in many ways a replica of this world, complete with the same social organization, is something that has not escaped the attention of well-known students of African thought. It is not clear, however, that the conceptual implications of this replication have been grasped. On the other hand, if the doctrine of immortality to be compared to its general African counterpart is the resurrection of the body, then there are certainly some analogies though, as can be expected, they are limited.

Another important difference between the Akan concept of *okra* and neo-Cartesian concepts of the soul is that in the latter, the soul is also the mind; in the former, *okra* is the life principle as distinct from the mind. The *okra* may perhaps have a mind, but it is not the mind in the Akan view. Mind is not a kind of entity, spiritual or otherwise, but a capacity to think and act in various ways based on states and processes of the brain (*amene*).[15] The mind is, in Akan doctrine, a most important component of personhood. The entire exposition of the normative component of personhood, which occupied us in the first half of this paper, was nothing but an exposition on the mind as an aspect of personhood. It was not an ontological account on the nature of the mind but on its social meaning; the concept of a person is a social concept before it is anything else.

One may therefore sum up the Akan doctrine of personhood by saying that a person consists of the life principle, the blood principle, the mind, and the charisma principle, and if these are in equilibrium, the subject is in good health. If the subject is not in good health, the chances are that more than one component is out of balance. This is the view that guides an Akan traditional healer who, when confronted with a sick patient, will almost invariably explore the hypothesis of psychological factors arising from social dislocations as a root cause of the malady at hand.

NOTES

1. This is not, however, to deny that some English speaking thinkers have developed social theories of personhood. Recall for example, George Herbert Mead's theory in his *Mind Self and Society* (Chicago: Chicago University Press, 1934). The point made in the text is the meanings of the relevant words in ordinary speech.

2. See for example, M. Fortes, "The Political System of the Tallensi of the Northern Territories of the Gold Coast" in *African Political Systems*, ed. M. Fortes and E. E. Evans-Pritchard (Oxford: Oxford University Press, 1940). Speaking of the Tallensi, Fortes asserts, "They had, in short, no 'tribal' government. . . " (p. 241). Evans-Pritchard, also writing on "The Nuer of the Southern Sudan" in the same volume, says, "In the strict sense of the word, the Nuer have no law. There is no one with legislative or juridical functions" (p. 293) and "if the Nuer has no law, likewise he lacks government" (p. 294).

3. See further Kwasi Wiredu, "An Akan Perspective on Human Rights" in *Human Rights in Africa: Cross-Cultural Perspectives* ed. Abdullahi Ahmed An-Naim and Francis M. Deng (Washington, D.C.: Brookings Institution, 1990).

4. I use the word "soul" here for lack of a better word, as will shortly be revealed.

5. Exceptional cases are not unknown, however, in which an individual, making outstanding contributions to society at lineage and community levels in spite of irreparable physical impairment preventing procreation, has gained respect equivalent to that of personhood.

6. Note that "respectable" here indicates a level of respect beyond the basic respect to which every human being is entitled, by virtue simply of being a human being.

7. C. A. Akrofi in his *Twi Mmebusem: Twi Proverbs* (Kumasi, Ghana: Presbyterian Book Depot and London: Macmillan and Co. Ltd., 1958) explains this name and the origin of this particular formulation of the proverb as follows. Birebire, the wife of Ntim Gyakari, a historical king of Dankyira, an Akan state, went to Adanse, another Akan state, and got seduced by Antwi, a royal person of Adanse. The latter, on discovery, was promptly executed, provoking the thought that if the lady had not come along, the tragic temptation would not have wrought its effect.

8. What is thought to affect free will is the special causation involved in unfavorable predestination or victimization by extrahuman forces.

9.   See the reprint of chapter 7 of Schlick's "Problems of Ethics" in *A Modern Introduction to Philosophy*, ed. Paul Edwards and Arthur Pap (New York: Free Press, 1973), 3rd ed.

10.   The two papers of Hospers referred to here are "Free will and Psychoanalysis," first published in *Philosophy and Phenomenological Research* (1950) and reprinted in *A Modern Introduction to Philosophy*; and "What means This Freedom?" in *Determinism and Freedom in an Age of Modern Science*, ed. Sidney Hook (New York: Collier Books, 1961).

11.   For the sake of simplicity, I have ignored horizontal complications. Since at any one time there are a number of spheres of conduct in each of which one might be going up or down "the person/nonperson" ladder, any comparison of the overall levels of two individuals or one individual at different times could be quite a tricky mathematical problem.

12.   See, for example, W. E. Abraham, *The Mind of Africa* (Chicago: University of Chicago Press, 1962), 60.

13.   K. A. Busia, "The Ashanti" in *African Worlds: Studies in the Cosmological Ideas and Social Values of African Peoples* ed. Daryll Forde (Oxford: Oxford University Press, 1954), 197.

14.   See also Kwasi Wiredu, "Death and the Afterlife in African Culture" in *Perspectives on Death and Dying: Cross-Cultural and Multi-Disciplinary Views*, ed. Arthur Berger et. al. (Philadelphia: The Charles Press, 1989).

15.   Here also see Kwasi Wiredu, "The Concept of Mind with Particular Reference to the Language and Thought of the Akans" in *African Philosophy*, vol 5 of *Contemporary Philosophy: A New Survey*, ed. G. Floistad (Boston: Kluwer Academic Publishers, 1987).

LAURENCE THOMAS

The Morally Beautiful

A remarkable affinity exists, I believe, between female and African-American experience. At heart, both traditions take seriously the importance of being morally constituted through the other. I also believe that healing—whether physical, spiritual, or moral—is more likely to occur if the persons seeking it are affirmed by others. It is unfortunate, therefore, that the effort to thrive in an oppressive society can also lead African-Americans to disregard an important social asset, namely, a regard for the other in moral development.

In fact, ethical egoism and Kantian ethics constitute radically different and incompatible moral traditions. Speaking rather freely, one could say that each tradition is a source of criticism of the other: egoism reminds us that Kantian ethics loses something important in its extreme other-regarding conception; Kantian ethics, that egoism loses something important in its extreme self-centeredness. But, while each tradition is critiqued by the other, the criticisms, like the traditions from which they begin, travel independently of one another.

As no line of argument has been suggested that is at once a criticism of egoism and Kantian ethics, perhaps no such argument is to be had. On the other hand, the trade-off between the two traditions suggests that each shares an underlying text or theme. I understand that theme to be about the metaphysics of the moral self, that is, about the way in which the self is morally constituted. The exploration of this theme, in female and African-American experience, will, in my opinion, identify it as a criticism of both traditions.

I am inspired by Carol Gilligan's discussion of abortion and women's self-conceptions in her important work, *In a Different Voice*.[1]

She speaks of themes to which all women can relate. As a caveat, let me say that I do not make the strong claim that Gilligan would actually endorse the account I am offering. But she need not do that in order for me to have been truly inspired by her.

WITHOUT DELIBERATE CHOICE

Women can become pregnant. And even outside the context of rape, their doing so need not be a matter of choice: "I want to become pregnant, so let me . . ." Contraceptives can fail; and in moments of heightened passion, the consequences of pregnancy may weigh less heavily on one—something to be thought about later. Whatever the case, to be a woman is to be profoundly aware of the reality that one's being pregnant need not be a matter of deliberate choice. In becoming pregnant, a woman is obviously faced with an enormous moral responsibility; and this is so even if she should choose to have an abortion. She can choose to come to terms with the child, or she can choose to have an abortion. She must choose, however. And the choice is morally significant, regardless of how she chooses. The moral responsibility for the choice she makes falls on no one else.

To be a woman, then, is to live with the reality that one may have a significant moral responsibility that one simply did not choose to have.[2] Although men can cause pregnancy without deliberate choice, pregnancy does not inform the moral reality of men in the same way as it does for women, since coming to terms with the fetus or aborting it does not involve the male's body. Men can run away from pregnancy; women cannot.

As is well known, those considerations inspire the idea that women and men operate within different moral frameworks, and with different ways of conceiving the moral self: women embrace the moral ideal that persons can have significant moral responsibility that they have not chosen, whereas men embrace the moral ideal that they have significant moral responsibility only if they have chosen it. The morality of men is definitive only of their rational choices; the morality of women is definitive of their rational choices and unchosen responsibility. I will refer to these two frameworks as the "responsibility" and the "choice" frameworks, respectively.

Now, straightaway, Gilligan's work invites the thought that there is a moral point of view of fundamental significance, which is accessible to women, but utterly inaccessible to men—at least not accessible to men without great difficulty, since there is no masculine experience to which it can be anchored, there being no male analogue to pregnancy. The point is not that women have a moral good that men lack—all kinds of people have moral goods that others lack—but that women have, in virtue of being women, a profound kind of indispensable moral understanding or outlook such that men cannot have in virtue of being men.

I shall not speculate on what a careful and thorough reading of Gilligan's work would deliver regarding this issue, though I would hope that her work yields the view that women do not have a moral framework inaccessible to men. Instead, I shall argue independently that this is not the case. The responsibility framework has, so I shall argue, a deep hold on all of us, even if there are differences between women and men on this score. There is nothing at all untoward about this last remark. After all, although all healthy and fully developed people have the capacity to express themselves in a natural language, we nonetheless think it perfectly plausible to hold that some have a gift for such expression, from which it is not thought to follow in the least that those who are not so gifted suffer from some defect or disorder.

THE CHILD SIDE OF MORAL EXPERIENCE

The human experience that gives the responsibility moral framework a hold on all of us is the child side of the parent-child relationship. When this relationship is as it should be, parents love their children, and this love is unmistakably clear in the mind of the child. The constants of physical displays and verbal expressions of affection, coupled with emotional comfort and support, suffice to secure in a child the deep conviction that he or she is truly loved by the parents. As is well-known, the child is immensely responsive to parental love, forms profoundly deep ties of affection, and so comes to love its parents, as a result of their continually manifesting their love for him or her. This fact is no doubt obvious; but the obvious, in this instance, must not go unappreciated.

The claim that the child comes to love its loving parents does not express a indeterminate feature of normal and healthy child development in the way that, for example, becoming left-or right-handed does. A child's coming to love his or her parents in return for their love is part of psychologically healthy child development. Loving parents may have a child who becomes left-handed, or instead, right-handed. Psychological theory does not yield strong conclusions regarding the significance of parental love as a determining factor on this characteristic. In the same way, loving parents may have a child who takes an interest in mathematics rather than music or conversely. Again, psychological theory suggests that parental love does not favor either endeavor. But, when it comes to the child's being responsible to the love of its parents, psychological theory is absolutely unambiguous: the child should be responsive. There are no psychological considerations that allow for the possibility that a psychologically healthy child may be completely unresponsive to the love of its parents.

There are, to be sure, many psychological considerations that allow for unresponsiveness or warped responsiveness on the part of the child in the case of child abuse. Likewise, in the case of parents who do not know how to express adequately their love for the child. Perhaps the parents are overly stern, since they have a mistaken view about the role of sternness in a child's development. Psychological theory tells us that when the manifestation of parental love lacks constancy or is otherwise defeated, the child cannot be counted on to be responsive.

The significance of these considerations to males and females having access to the responsibility moral framework is this. To begin with, a child no more chooses to be an object of parental love than it chooses to be born. Second, a child does not choose to be responsive with love to the love of its parents. No, it comes to be responsive to their love. Responding with love is something that happens to a child. And, in no time, the child is no longer merely responsive to the parents' love, but also begins to express its love for its parents. The child smiles, kisses, and hugs them, for example. Of course, the child chooses to do these specific acts, but the intense feelings of love the child has toward its parents is not in any way chosen. The child's identification with its parents is not something that it chooses to have; nor likewise is the care and concern that the child comes to have for the well-being of its parents. Yet this response to love is a necessary part of the child's healthy psychological development.

What I specifically draw attention to is this: As our talk about the psychological development of the child in terms of responsiveness to its parents grows richer, the talk ineluctably has increasingly greater moral overtones. Two-year-olds love their parents, and by age eleven, care for them. They do not, however, choose to do either. Later, they begin to have a sense of appreciation for the sacrifices that their parents have made for them; but, again, they do not choose to have this sense of appreciation. And, finally, they develop deep feelings of gratitude for the many things that their parents have done for them. But, once more, they do not choose to have feelings of gratitude.

Feelings of gratitude are part of child development, given good parent-child relationships. Yet, gratitude is a moral notion. It requires having moral sensibilities to the efforts of others, and a willingness to acknowledge those efforts, at least occasionally, in both word and deed. While it is not clear that anyone can have a right to another's gratitude, the hold that gratitude can have on a person's life can be substantial—and rightly so. Why, we sometimes refuse deeds of genuine kindness in order to avoid the debt of gratitude, the sense that we are beholden to another. No such choice, however, is open to the child fortunate enough to have a good parent-child relationship.

It should be obvious, but is worth making explicit, and even repeating: moral sentiments—in particular, the moral sentiment of gratitude—have a hold on the child in virtue of normal, psychologically healthy development. Gender is not a factor here. There is a congruence between the psychological and the moral development of the child with respect to moral sentiments, which is the same for all children regardless of gender.[3] This claim is compatible with the position that, later, other things do make a difference in people's lives with respect to gender and the operation of the moral sentiments.

Obviously, having a deep sense of gratitude to one's parents is not, strictly speaking, identical to having some significant moral responsibility for them. It is possible to have one without the other. A child can be most grateful for all that his or her parents did for him, but if the parents should die when he or she is sixteen, then obviously two decades later, the child has no moral responsibility with respect to them, death-bed promises aside. I have not claimed, though, that gratitude and responsibility amount to the same thing. My point, rather, is that (a) feelings of gratitude toward one's parents can be extraordinarily deep; (b) such feelings operate irrespective of gender; (c) these feelings are not chosen; and (d) such feelings of gratitude allow that one's parents have a claim on one—a claim that one did not choose that they have. This claim is close to, but not identical to, the claim that a child has an unchosen moral responsibility to its parents.

The claim is close enough, surely, to suppose that in its wake comes accessibility to the responsibility moral framework. For the hold that gratitude has on us is by no means trivial, as is shown by the fact that we sometimes resist being in a position to owe gratitude to another.

There is yet another point that will serve us well as the argument proceeds, namely, the role that parental affirmation plays in the life of the child.

Clearly, no child learns to interact effectively with its environment, and so to perform various tasks efficiently and skillfully simply by being told what to do. Instruction, though necessary, is hardly sufficient. The support and the encouragement that the child receives are absolutely indispensable. No child learns to tie shoes, for example, simply by being shown how to do it, and then being told by a stern voice to do it. This task, done mindlessly by most adults, is rather daunting to a child. Again, most adults give no thought to cutting their food before they eat. But for even a bright child this mundane task seems quite formidable. It is a question of holding the fork in the right way and holding the knife in the right way; then placing both on the food in the right way; then bearing down just the right amount; and moving the knife back and forth in the right way. What the adult sees as one task, the child sees as several that have to be co-ordinated just so. The fact that a child learns to cut food with a knife and fork at all, is because he or she has been shown how to do it, been allowed to make mistakes, been praised for each bit of progress, and further encouraged.

At the very heart of parental affirmation is the child's trust in its parents. Most important, it is not because the child is affirmed by its parents that it trusts them; rather it is because the child trusts them that it is affirmed by them. For while positive judgments affirm the child and buoys its spirit, negative judgments are a blow to its self-esteem. The child is vulnerable to its parents in this way: it can be affirmed by what they say only if it can also be disconfirmed by what they say.

These remarks complete our discussion of the child aspect of the parent-child relationship, and the endeavor to show that as a result of this relationship, everyone has access to the moral responsibility framework. I want now to show, in the order mentioned, the applications of these considerations to ethical egoism and Kantian ethics.

THE CASE AGAINST EGOISM AND KANTIAN ETHICS

Ethical egoism maintains that each person should regard the self and only the self as an end per se. All others have only instrumental value. But being an ethical egoist cannot be easy. Specifically, it is manifestly clear, given our account of child development, that the healthy psychological development of the child is most incongruous with ethical egoism. The child's sense of gratitude to its parents simply cannot be explicated in terms of egoism. The child does not feel gratitude in order to maximize its self-interest, even if its feelings happen to yield precisely this result.

It may be thought that the adult can put off the claims of childhood and that ethical egoism, though not for the child, is congruous with the psychology of the adult. But the psychology of the self is far too continuous for any such claim to be true. A few reflections can serve to bolster this straightforward response.

To be an ethical egoist is to take only oneself as an end in itself. But even an ethical egoist must make judgments concerning the endeavors of one's own self, and it is not clear that this can be done without reference to others. The ethical egoist's judgment about doing well or performing the right tasks cannot be made independently of others. Rather, from time to time the ethical egoist must look to others to underwrite self-assessment. The problem of trust raises its mighty head.

First, another's judgment that one performs a certain activity well—playing the piano, for example—can be affirming only if one values the judgment of that person. It is one thing for an Andre Watts or a Leonard Bernstein to offer this judgment and quite another for a vagabond getting off the subway. Still, not even a compliment from Bernstein will be affirming if one does not value his opinion in the first place. That is, the judgment is not affirming just because one needs a compliment from someone and Bernstein happens to be in the area. The valuing of anyone's opinion cannot be simply instrumental in nature: one needs a comment from Bernstein, so one values it.

Second, a compliment from Bernstein will affirm the ethical egoist only if one trusts his positive assessment to be sincere. But, as we saw in our discussion of child-development, if a sincere positive judgment would affirm the ethical egoist, then a sincere negative one would be disconfirming and a blow to self-esteem. Needless to say, if these things are true, then it is not at all obvious to what extent the egoist can take only the self as an end in itself, unless others are taken as ends in themselves. But most assuredly this move is the ethical egoist's undoing.

Kantian ethics, on the other hand, places a premium on free and rational choice. It maintains that we constitute ourselves as moral creatures by making free and rational choices. This claim would perhaps be defensible were it not that Kantian ethics seems to entail that we cannot be morally constituted in any other way. This very strong claim is manifestly false. The story of child-development told above makes this demonstrably clear. The gratitude which the child feels toward its parents is a deep feature of the child's life that cannot be explained as a result of choice. It is a truth that the child is morally constituted; it is a falsehood that it is constituted as a result of free and rational choice. The child is morally constituted through the other—its parents in this case. That we are morally constituted through the other does not cease to be so, even if later on the continuation of our moral constitution requires choice. At any rate, Kantians have given us no reason to think that it does cease to be so. The best evidence, however, that we remain morally constituted through others is the role that moral affirmation plays in our lives.

THE MARK OF MORAL FLOURISHING

Nothing better replenishes the energy we expend living morally than affirmation from others. If one has risked one's life to save another; if one has given until it hurts (and this becomes a matter of public knowledge); if one has been particularly outspoken for the cause of right, thereby jeopardizing one's career—if one has done any of these things, nothing better strengthens one's resolve to continue doing right than moral affirmation. We draw strength constantly from the expressions of appreciation, gratitude, or admiration of others.

An act of duty done solely for the sake of duty can never be as morally affirming as an act of duty done out of love, and the difference is substantial. To be sure, it can in some instances be better to have an act done merely out of duty than not to have it done at all. In terms of moral affirmation, however, such an act does not begin to approach the affirmation that comes in the wake of an act of duty done out of love.

Acts of moral affirmation are acts that issue from a highly commendable moral attitude, which explains why they fall into the category of the moral—a category not exhausted by duties, rights, and obligations. And this attitude constitutes not just a commitment to doing what is right, since one can be quite parsimonious with respect to that commitment, but an attitude of good will, generosity, and kindness toward others. Acts of moral affirmation empower and enliven us. They are morally beautiful in their own right.

To be human is to be constituted by the other both intellectually and emotionally. It would be stunning if morality were the exception. The claim that we are quintessentially social creatures should be understood in this light.

Kantians would say that the mark of moral flourishing is not found in anything but choice. But that is not the case. Our moral flourishing is inescapably tied to our being vulnerable in ways that make it possible for others to affirm us, not because they are required to, but because they care—which is why friendships and love are so important in our lives. Yet, as important as affirmation is to our flourishing, it really takes very little to affirm us. Therein lies the beauty.

A final comment: much social interaction is anchored in nonverbal behavior, and African-Americans are profoundly rich in their nonverbal skills, as people often are who have been through forms of oppression which radically discount, at least officially, their moral and intellectual skills. We could be masters at affirming one another, if only we wanted to be. And this would make us richer human beings—and better—physically, spiritually, and morally.

The Kantian framework makes free choice an ontologically prior aspect of the moral landscape. If our account of moral development is sound, that framework is in fact false. What is prior is our moral sensibilities. And it is this truth that, I think, resonates profoundly with African-American experience. But, as often happens among the oppressed, we have lost sight of our own gifts.

NOTES

1. Carol Gilligan, *In a Different Voice* (Cambridge: Harvard University Press, 1982).

2. Of course, some women are born—or become—sterile, and all women, if they should live long enough, move beyond childbearing years. But, the force of the argument is not defeated by these considerations. For it is very rare that a woman knows that she is sterile from adolescence on. And women beyond childbearing years have, nonetheless, lived with the moral reality that I have described.

3. Lawrence Kohnberg makes a similar claim, bur from a very different perspective. His claim is about cognitive moral development. See his "Essays in Moral Development," in *The Philosophy of Moral Development: Moral Stages and the Idea of Justice* I (New York: Harper and Row, 1981). For a critique, see my "Moral and Psychological Development," in *A Companion to Ethics*, ed. Peter Singer (Oxford: Basil Blackwell, publication pending).

J. Bryan Hehir:

Responses to
Kwasi Wiredu and
Laurence Thomas

My assigned task is to respond to two papers, Professor Wiredu's "The African Concept of Personhood," and Professor Thomas's "The Morally Beautiful." It is also necessary to indicate that Professor Wiredu's paper is based on his other contribution to this symposium, entitled, "The Moral Foundations of African Culture." Having set forth the assignment, I should say a word about the limits of the respondent. I am neither a philosopher nor an expert on African or African-American culture; my background is in Catholic theological ethics and in international politics. My participation in the program is based less on previous exposure to the themes of the two papers than on the inveterate habit I have developed of responding affirmatively to Ed Pellegrino's requests—who in multiple ways daily enriches our lives.

Having exposed my vulnerabilities, I will now indicate how I have tried to compensate for them. The method is straightforward: I will discuss what I know and seek intersection with the themes of the two papers assigned to me. The connection is not artificial. As I read the papers, particularly Professor Wiredu's contributions, I was struck by the comparable themes that exist between the African (i.e., the Akan) concepts of personhood and society and basic themes in Catholic social thought. Consequently my response to the papers will have two parts: I will first sketch the substance and structure of Catholic social teaching that is comparable to the Wiredu and Thomas papers; then I will indicate points of convergence and identify questions which arise from a comparison of Catholic concepts and those used in the two papers.

CATHOLIC SOCIAL ETHICS

Within the limits imposed by time and the genre of a response to the contribution of others, I will sketch the character of Catholic social ethics and its structural categories. Essentially, Catholic social teaching is a religiously grounded ethic which is articulated principally in philosophical rather than theological terms. The sources of the social ethic are the biblical resources of revelation and the philosophical categories of reason. The biblical roots, the Jewish and Christian scriptures, establish the foundation and perspectives of the social ethic. The biblical categories are interpreted authoritatively by the teaching office of the Church. Although these religious roots of the social ethic are pervasively present in its development and articulation, they often do not appear in an explicit way. The ethic, designed to address a range of social questions that affect the Church and the wider society, is cast primarily in the concepts and language of Natural Law social philosophy.

The Natural Law ethic predated Christianity but has been used extensively in Catholic teaching as a means of mediating the religiously-based categories of the tradition, relating them to specific political, legal, economic, and international issues. The ethic is derived through rational reflection on human nature and experience, seeking to answer two questions: "What is a human person?" and "What is the person's relationship to society?" In the words of John Courtney Murray, the natural law ethic seeks "to give a philosophical account of the moral experience of humanity and to lay down a charter of essential humanism" (*We Hold These Truths* [New York: Sheed & Ward, 1960], p. 297).

As developed in Catholic social teaching, the Natural Law social ethic is based on a conception of the dignity of the human person. The person, understood theologically as the *imago dei*, is understood philosophically as a creature of transcendent worth, distinguished from the rest of the created order by a capacity for rational reflection and free choice. The person, in the words of Pope Pius XII (ca. 1958), is the subject, the foundation, and the end of the social order. The significance of this proposition is that every social system—political, economic, or legal—will be judged by how it protects or fails to protect human dignity.

In light of its conception of the person, the Natural Law ethic develops a theory of human rights and duties, moral claims, and moral obligations that are rooted in human nature and articulated over time. Rights in this tradition are understood as moral claims which can be immunities (political and civil rights) or empowerments (social and economic rights). Rights are correlated with duties; each person possesses rights and duties; one person's right imposes on another a duty to respect and respond to that right.

This conception of rights and duties is rooted in a definition of the social nature of the person. In the Natural Law tradition the person is social by nature, not by choice. The person belongs by nature to three communities: the family, civil society, and the human community. Much of Natural Law social teaching is directed toward establishing norms for structuring these three communities. The emphasis in Catholic teaching on the social nature of the person sets it off from more individualistic liberal theories on the relationship of the person and society.

More specifically, both the organic conception of society and the positive (if still limited) role of the state found in Catholic teaching distinguish its social philosophy from social contract theories and from a view that the state's role is exhausted by its function of maintaining domestic order and providing for the defense of society.

Finally, the general social theory outlined in this Natural Law conception yields four areas of applied ethics: (1) a theory of jurisprudence which holds that positive law and policy are always subject to evaluation by the unwritten "higher" moral law; (2) a sexual ethic; (3) a medical ethic; and (4) an ethic of international relations.

RELATING DIFFERENT TRADITIONS

I find three points of comparison between themes found in the Wiredu and Thomas papers and the ideas I have just summarized.

The first is the relationship of religious belief and moral norms. Professor Wiredu, in his paper, "The Moral Foundations of African Culture," describes "the independence of morality from religion in the Akan outlook." He then goes on to the assertion that, "the will of God, not to talk of any other extrahuman being, is logically incapable of defining the good." In these two statements are both convergence and divergence with a Catholic conception of the sources of moral knowledge.

On the one hand, there is at least an analogy in the distinction between religion and morality to the Catholic understanding that there are two sources of moral wisdom, viz., biblical revelation and rational norms derived from an understanding of human nature. Rather than a complete dichotomy of religion and morality as the Wiredu position states the case, the Catholic style is to distinguish the two forms of moral argument, but to see them ultimately as complementary.

The commandments, for example, found in both the Jewish and Christian scriptures, are regarded as specifying the moral truths embedded in the Natural Law. The complementarity of revelation and reason in turn distinguishes the Catholic from the Akan position on Professor Wiredu's point that the "the will of God" cannot define the good. The Catholic tradition (with some exceptions) would agree that a voluntarist conception of the good is inadequate to relate revelation and reason. But an intellectualist conception of the good can establish the foundation of the moral order in the mind of God. It would then see God as revealing the moral order directly through revelation and mediately through human nature. Professor Wiredu has made a strong point of the fact that both religion and morality are solidly intellectual in the Akan tradition. But he does not pursue the question of whether an intellectual grounding of good and right could unite the spheres of religion and morality.

To summarize the Catholic and the Akan positions on the source of morality, there is a formal similarity in seeking to distinguish religion and morality, but the Akan position separates the two more absolutely than the Catholic position does, and the Akan position seems to conceive of the possible relationship of God and the moral life only in voluntarist terms, a position that it then rejects. The dominant Catholic position would also reject this view, but then conceive of the relationship of religion and morality on a different basis wherein faith enhances and expands the horizon of reason, but also grounds the moral order in the divine intellect.

The second point of comparison is more direct and complementary than the first. It concerns the conception of the human person and the basis of human dignity. In his paper, "The African Concept of Personhood," Professor Wiredu says, "the Akans hold that there is a divine element in the nature of all human beings. On this ground alone, everyone, young or old, is entitled to a certain minimum of respect and dignity and a full complement of human rights." This response has already commented on the centrality of the human person in both personal and social Catholic moral teaching. The centrality of the teaching is tied to the moral status of the person as understood by revelation and reason. While the philosophical argument distinguishes the person from the rest of the created order on the basis of intelligence and freedom, the theological view goes further, describing the person as the *imago dei*, the clearest reflection of God in all creation.

The theological position corresponds closely with Professor Wiredu's notion of a "divine element" in human nature. More specifically, the theological view deepens the philosophical judgment about the spiritual nature of the person in two ways. First, the distinguishing human capacities of intellect and will in fact reflect the dynamism of the inner life of the Trinity where Father, Son, and Spirit are related in terms of knowledge and love. Second, the doctrine of the Incarnation (the central Christian revelation that God became man in the person of his Son, Jesus Christ) provides new meaning to the concept of human dignity. Because Christ assumed a human nature joined to a divine personality, Christian teaching holds that every person who shares human nature now has a new bond and relationship with God. These religious themes, *imago dei* and the Incarnation, are not meant to diminish the significance of the philosophical view of the human person. Following the perspective developed above on the sources of moral knowledge, the theological arguments are designed to build on and enhance the insights of reason. It is in this sense that Thomas Aquinas argued that grace perfects nature; the "divine element," to use Professor Wiredu's phrase, consecrates that which reason has already honored by its assessment of human dignity.

The third point of comparison is the social nature of the person. Both the Wiredu papers and Professor Thomas's paper, "The Morally Beautiful," affirm a concept of the person which fits substantially the Catholic philosophical anthropology undergirding its social teaching. The main theme of Professor Thomas's paper, as I read it, is "about the metaphysics of the moral self, that is, the way in which the self is morally constituted." In criticizing both egoism and a Kantian view of ethics, Professor Thomas urges us to take "seriously the import of being morally constituted through the other." He goes on to specify this perspective: "To be human is to be constituted by the other both emotionally and intellectually." I do not think this idea could be so strongly stated in Catholic thought; to say that we are "constituted" through others seems to erode too much the concept of a "subsistent being," which is at the core of a Catholic conception of personhood. But the relational concept of the person that Thomas argued finds a reflection in the strong social notions of personality and morality that run through Catholic ethics.

Catholic thinking on personhood is characterized by a conception of the person as existing at the heart of a social fabric in a web of personal and social relationships flowing from human nature. This makes it quite compatible with what Professor Wiredu described as "the deeply communalistic conception of human existence entertained among the peoples of Africa." The compatibility is evident in two of the implications that Professor Wiredu draws from his social conception of the person. First, as he puts it, "a human being is social before he or she is political." I found this statement correct and I would only say it is then extended in Catholic teaching to say that because the person is social, the society must be "political," that is, be organized in terms of political authority expressed in and through a state. The state's authority is limited by the moral claims of the person, the higher claims of religion, and the limited but real social role of other associations in society. Second, Professor Wiredu makes the point that rights and duties are correlative concepts, developed in light of the several social responsibilities which test the moral standing of the person. Both the social conception of rights and duties and their correlative relationship find echoes in Catholic social philosophy. There is some difference, I believe, on the point Professor Wiredu makes in his paper between the ontological status of a human being, and the further moral tests one must successfully meet to be regarded as truly a person. This distinction in Catholic thought would be expressed by saying that every human being is truly a person but that the moral character of a person is something shaped by the pursuit of virtue.

By isolating these three notions from the Wiredu and Thomas papers, I have tried to demonstrate analogous conceptions of personal and social morality between Catholic and Akan thought. The analogy, as always, admits of similitude and significant difference, but given the quite different presuppositions of the two systems, the elements of commonality are significant. Christian thought, and particularly its sub-system of Catholic thought, are cast in universal categories. Nevertheless, it takes a work of discernment and articulation to relate the Christian corpus to diverse philosophical systems. Preliminary indications from the papers to which I am responding indicate significant possibilities for development.

Further questions would need to be explored, among them the following: (1) how the teaching of rights and duties would be played out in Akan thought; (2) how the social and political, distinguished by Professor Wiredu, are to be related; and (3) how both Akan ethics and the relational-responsibility ethic used by Professor Thomas would take shape in areas of applied ethics (sexual, medical, and social), which are so large a part of Catholic moral teaching. This is a task, however, for an independent paper, not a response.

LEONARD HARRIS

Autonomy Under Duress

"What is the nature of health or wellness from an African-American perspective?" "What are the roles of healers and patients in African and African-American cultures?" These questions suggest certain answer types. The first question presupposes a phenomenon, "health," on which African-Americans have a particular perspective. "Health," suggests at least one of the following answers: either "health" is intended to indicate a broad range of related phenomena or an essence of such phenomena. If an individual, or African people in general, hold ideas similar to the materialism of Hobbes, for example, they might believe that health means proper mechanistic or, in modern terms, neurological functioning of the body.

But there are other possibilities: Kantians, for example, may believe that health is the continuity of embodied transcendental consciousness; absolute idealists, that it is a congruence of a self-identified consciousness operating in an idealized domain. Among pragmatists, health may be construed as the existence of embodied experience in ways that allow for enriching instrumental manipulation of the environment; teleological determinists—Edward Wilmot Blyden, for example—may believe that health is the embodiment of "kind" or race purity living in accordance with its nature; and, lastly, Akan believers may conceive of health in terms of a peaceful embodied spirit.

The elements of this short list of possible beliefs from which to develop a detailed conception of health share an important feature: each recommends either a metaphysical or transcendental essence that is encoded in our being, of whose essence, individuals can be instances. Thus, the existence of healthy persons is the instantiation of the ontological nature of humans as mediated by, or in congruence with, their metaphysical or transcendental essence. The relationship between patient and physician or healer would on these accounts be constructed or prescribed according to some modality that best promotes the realization of our ontological being.

The World Health Organization (WHO) avoids expressed commitment to metaphysical or transcendental beliefs. WHO's definition of health focuses on the ontological character of persons. And because it is a broad definition of health that is constantly debated and critiqued, it has progressively changed. It now incorporates conceptions of the patient as an autonomous agent and of health care professionals as equal rather than paternal agents of the mental and physical well-being of patients.

I will argue that concepts of autonomy do not escape entrapment in a web of meaning, that is, epistemological figures and intervening background assumptions that shape how subjects are constructed as agents. Concepts of autonomy allow for special criteria applicable to differentiated groups, for example, children or mentally impaired persons. Identical physiologies, however, as my examples will indicate, can be seen as categorically different depending on how subjects are constructed. Although a good deal of emphasis is usually placed on the existence of biological differences, comparatively little attention has focused on biological identities that are perceived as categorically different, depending on how the subject is constructed. Procedures for reasoning from principles or concepts to practice, inclusive of criteria for revising judgments to prevent prejudice, are, I argue, incomplete in ways that tend to ignore the importance of background assumptions. The idea I argue for is that there are limits for what we can expect a concept, even a theoretically rich concept, of autonomous persons to provide. I will suggest that at least one feature of African-American history—the tradition that critiques and struggles against dominant authorities within the health care system—often compels revaluation of background assumptions.

By "autonomy" I will mean one of two views: (a) that autonomy is a form of independence and authenticity; that a person's preferences are to be honored if they accord with what he or she chooses or would choose under normal conditions; (b) that autonomy is a form of independence; it is also a side constraint such that a principle of respect for persons or bodily integrity may outweigh a person's preference, even if such preferences are in accord with their authenticity under normal conditions.[1] These views of autonomy are rule-governed. That is, they define autonomy (independence, authenticity), conditions for its effective expression (honor free choice, authenticity; respect for persons outweighing authenticity), and reasoning procedures for its appropriate application. There are certainly other views of autonomy besides these two and a wide range of reasoning procedures that can be applied. I believe, however, that these two views are strong, rule-governed approaches associated with theoretically rich reasoning procedures, and particularly well-developed Kantian deontological, contractarian, or utilitarian procedures.

THE PATIENT DR. DICK DID NOT FAIL TO SEE

There once was a physician named Dr. Dick, a good doctor who was, by popular accounts, also a good person. That is, he was inclined to evaluate his cases strenuously and on rationally ethical principles, whether or not so doing was a requirement of his profession. He was an ardent admirer of Ralph Waldo Emerson, taking particular delight in Emerson's *Self Reliance, Nature,* and *Nominalist & Realist.* And, like most physicians, Dr. Dick was a realist. He usually considered deontological standpoints, utilitarian calculations, contractarian sensibilities, and his religious feelings in formulating ethical beliefs. He steadfastly tried to avoid logical errors in reasoning from beliefs to practices regardless of which standpoint he was testing prior to finally deciding. Since each standpoint was itself regarded as a rational mode of arriving at defensible actions, his survey approach offered a reasonable chance of acting justly.

Dr. Dick was concerned with the welfare of his community. He offered advice to patients on how to prevent illness. He studied diligently to remain abreast of new and well-tested cures. He treated patients as rational and autonomous agents, as best he understood what these terms entailed. He made sure that his patients were informed about available treatments, treatment options, known and possible effects. In cases in which the best interest of a patient was not served by the patient's choice of therapy, he required extensive counseling, but in the end he tended to defer to a patient's will as long as it did not conflict with his view of respect for bodily integrity or authenticity. (He never confronted cases that involved a conflict between respect for integrity and authenticity, i.e., cases in which integrity demanded a cure that traditions of authenticity required rejecting.) In cases that seemed open to conflicting actions, he relied on other experts or the direction his good intentions recommended.

Dr. Dick believed that all persons regardless of race, religion, creed, gender, or nationality were equal members of the human family, endowed by their creator with inalienable rights. In this belief he differed radically from other members of his community, medical profession, religion, and social network; nonetheless, as a good person, he persevered in his belief. He charged blacks and whites alike according to their ability to pay and services rendered, as well as, I might add, contributing his services once weekly, free of charge, to persons unable to pay.

Dr. Dick specialized in castration and abortion. As it happened one day, Dr. Dick made George Washington Carver a eunuch.

Dr. Dick had evaluated the practice of castration for the purpose of making eunuchs. He concluded that it was ethically justifiable according to several well-reasoned theories. On utilitarian grounds, his patients would become highly-valued house servants and accountants. As house servants, they would likely receive some education and better treatment than field hands. They would avoid being lynched because they would be incapable of rape, given the type of castrations Dr. Dick performed. Although approximately 26 percent of lynchings in the United States had to do with accusations of rape, Dr. Dick was acutely aware of the popular practice of lynching. If a eunuch were accused of looking at a white woman the wrong way, at most he would probably receive a stout beating but not be lynched.[2]

Eunuchs normally held much higher status than slaves. They were natally alienated absolutely: they could not procreate or adopt; therefore, their kinship links were severed.[3] Their existence was strictly confined to being dedicated subordinates—a dedication enhanced by the impossibility of participating in creating progeny. Universally despised, unable to constitute a class to command power across kinship or generations, and bereft of the possibility of willing property to immediate biological family, eunuchs were prized possessions connoting a master's tremendous wealth.

By castration, therefore, George Washington Carver would become, to some degree, deracinated, i.e., no longer a Negro capable of procreating and perpetuating the race but a titular-free surrogate, dedicated to service, and incapable of shaping a personally connected ascension of progeny. Dr. Dick reasoned that the young Carver would be fortunate to have the opportunity to express his genuine, or authentic, character under the improved conditions that "eunuchization" offered. Dr. Dick felt that he was constrained from making eunuchs of those for whom nature or circumstance was incongruous with the condition, and that he could not in good conscience refuse to act to offer a therapeutic benefit.

On deontological grounds, Dr. Dick felt that the integrity of a eunuch's body was preserved because informed consent was required prior to castration. Independent of consent, Dr. Dick reasoned, that if we were Carver with Carver's limited options, life chances, cultural specificity, and natural passions, it would not be unreasonable for us to choose castration. Moreover, the practice of castration for the purpose of making eunuchs was an ancient practice in nearly all systems of slavery. On Christian and Judaic grounds, the good doctor was apprised by received tradition that scripture did not strictly forbid making eunuchs of those destined for service, particularly if there were reasons to believe that their souls might thereby have a better chance of salvation.

Dr. Dick sold excised penises and testacies, or, as he preferred to call them, excised organs, to local stores for display or to wealthy white women as decorative ornaments and conversation pieces. He always sought permission from donors, shared the profit with the donors, and contributed to a local charity from his share of the profit. The historical record does not tell us what he did with Carver's penis, but it does tell us what procedures Dr. Dick followed before consenting to operate.

Dr. Dick discussed the operation extensively with Carver's master, his guardians (because he was an orphan), and with Carver himself. The master, it seems, needed a new house servant and companion for his daughter. Dr. Dick thought his reasons were too paternalistic. Carver's guardians, contrary to the normal practice of other physicians, were consulted. They consented on grounds that it would offer a better life for him. Although Dr. Dick knew that the consent was made under duress, he nonetheless considered the reason a strong one. Eleven-year-old Carver, again contrary to popular practices, was also consulted. The youth wanted to make everyone else happy and secure the opportunity for learning; he did not express a great interest in girls as future wives, but seemed ambivalent or uncertain about the prospects of losing his penis. Dr. Dick felt that young Carver's penis might be a cause of future trouble, and since it seemed that all parties involved had reflected on what Dr. Dick perceived as a therapeutic operation, therapeutic in the same way as Dr. Dick perceived abortions, he proceeded judiciously.

One way to understand Dr. Dick's approach to castration as therapeutic is to consider his approach to abortion. A fetus in a black woman's body, whether fertilized by a black or white male, was considered in Dr. Dick's society as fundamentally different from a fetus in a white woman's body. The black woman's fetus was potentially cheap labor, sex, and property. A white woman's fetus, if fertilized by a black male, represented pollution, disease, infection, and corruption. The first required a special argument to justify abortion—an argument that had to show benefit to the welfare of a white male or his family. The second demanded, required, and obviously warranted a cure, i.e., abortion on demand.

The privilege white women had to date rape black men, like the privilege white men had to date, wife, or slave rape, was well known but rarely acknowledged. A black male's refusal to be raped, or his participation in rape meant the possibility of facing dreaded accusations: that he looked licentious, made lewd gestures, suggested sexual contact, approached aggressively or even raped. Castration, lynching, and burning would be the probable reward reaped by a black male, and in some cases, by his wife and children. The punishment of lynching always occurred after ritual beating, limb decapitation, and the nationally practiced use of plunging a corkscrew into the body of blacks and reeling out flesh. Finally, parts of the corpse would be amputated as souvenirs for white men, women, and children.

The removal of a fetus from a white woman thought to have been fertilized by a black male was, for Dr. Dick, an unfortunate but necessary evil. He reasoned that neither the fetus nor the mother would live a flourishing life. The autonomy of the woman, as he constructed woman, was preserved. If the pregnancy was publicly known, the black father was probably already dead or a fugitive; if not publicly known, abortion might help prevent the father from being harmed. On deontological grounds, Dr. Dick reasoned that women were equal persons and had a fundamental right to bodily autonomy. It was inherently justifiable and utilitarian to perform abortions, he believed, and particularly so because the women he served were all white. The fetuses they wanted to abort were going to be Negroes, "octoroons," "quadroons," or some other dreaded category.

For Dr. Dick, the interracial fetus of a white woman held a similar status to that of a black male's penis—organs that could be justly excised after well-reasoned consent. Consent trumped utility, although such acts were further supported by utility; consent preserved freedom, independence, integrity, truthfulness, and the autonomy of agents as an inalienable good. Consent gained under duress was carefully weighed. Special attention was paid to whether the agent was well informed, to individual and social consequences, and to preserving authenticity, as these were understood and pertinent to the sort of agent involved.

I was told the following story by a poplar tree in Tuskegee, Alabama on September 7, 1980, my first day as the Portia-Washington-Pittman Fellow at Tuskegee Institute.

In a brief moment before the castration of young Carver, his matured soul, then inhabiting the body of an executive for the National Medical Association, migrated into his eleven-year-old body, the time warp allowing only a brief second of presence. That soul, whispered the tree, realizing what was happening although not empowered to do anything about it, yelled with murderous anger to Dr. Dick, "Whose damn life is it anyway?" Dr. Dick's adult soul, then inhabiting the body of an executive of the American Medical Association, had returned simultaneously and with the same time warp and power limitations to Dr. Dick's body. Realizing what was about to happen and hearing Carver's voice, Dr. Dick's soul with genuine frustration and regard, yelled back into the expanse of paraspace, "Yours." A faint echo, like a voice mix, was heard in the paraspace of the transcendental as the souls immediately resumed their matured spatial-temporal slots—"Ours." The moment passed.

This was the story of Dr. Dick's attitude toward the subject.[4]

In principle, Dr. Dick may not have objected to the castration of white males for the purpose of making them eunuchs. The possibility, however, of castrating whites did not fit the epistemological figures or background conceptions of subjects, that is, castration was too obviously not a benefit for whites, obviously in no one's interest, and obviously contrary to their natures, authenticity, traditions, integrity, and codes of honor. The fact that white males were not made eunuchs reflected social meanings; they were not, as agents, constituted as innately, irreversibly, and permanently subordinate persons. They were not natally alienated in the sense of being constructed as agents unable to define descending generations or control the direction of ascending generations. Moreover, the meaning of their independence, rationality, or authenticity was a function of the levels and types of intrinsic ontological merit they were assumed to represent.

Using the historical reality of "eunuchization" as a figurative example suggests that relevant facts about the body are constituted by virtue of what the body is as an objective entity enmeshed with meaning. As genealogical isolates, eunuchs represent the preservation of separateness over time. The possibility of affection, kinship, or family ties between master and subordinate are absolutely negated in them. Analogously, the constraints applied determining what would not be done to whites and what could be done to blacks was a function, not of the biological facts of identity, but of the way the body was constituted as different. The body of George Washington Carver, for example, belonged to Carver as agent, but the meaning of the agent's body was mediated by its social context. The bodily integrity of blacks was not violated, in Dr. Dick's view, because their integrity entailed living lives as subordinates, i.e., a fulfilling life for them was only possible as a life of happy or contented subordination. Their equality, in substance, meant a contentment that was equal in worth to the contentment of whites. The precondition for Dr. Dick to have arrived at a different view of person required a different set of intervening background assumptions about personhood, bodily integrity, the moral community, fulfilling lives and utility.

THE PATIENT DR. DEATH FAILED TO SEE

When I received the program from the Center for the Advanced Study of Ethics and learned that there would be two distinguished respondents to my paper—a paper that I had not completed writing—I was very apprehensive and considered several drastic options. I first considered calling the Center, feigning illness, and informing the Center that I would be regrettably unable to present my paper. I realized, however, that I would still be required to write and submit my paper, having previously agreed to do so. The respondents would still have a chance to critique my views, only I might be left in the dark about their critique; worse still, they might ignore my views and present contrary perspectives before an audience that might be otherwise receptive. Taking the option of feigning illness also meant that my honor as a promise-keeper would be compromised. Moreover, my utilitarian calculation of the consequences of failing to present suggested that it would cost me emotionally in ways I found basically unacceptable.

I next considered calling the Center and informing them that I was dead; but death normally includes the loss of the ability to communicate, at least over the telephone. Moreover, I would be lying if I were not dead. The option was rejected.

I then considered either presenting my paper and engaging in discussion and debate, or simply dying. I decided that it would be preferable to die rather than to live with any more apprehension, fail to be a promise-keeper when I was capable of keeping my promise, intentionally deceive, or risk having my views subjected to unanswered critique.

I called Dr. Death, who works at my HMO during the day and at the public hospital near my home on weekends. I spoke to Dr. Death's receptionist. Regardless of my urgent pleas, I was unable to get an appointment to see the good doctor in order to die until December. It was now August, and the program date was November

9. Dr. Death, it seems, had a long line of young African-American males, abused mothers, drug-addicted babies. Dr. Death had terror to inflict on the many African peoples whom Dr. Death's assistant, Dr. Misery, oppressed during their daily lives as powerless employees under the dominion of callous white males. Dr. Death stood at the hospital door, beckoning them in for treatment.

Dr. Death was overburdened as administrator for the maldistribution of public and private resources and too busy to insure that attention was paid to the doctor-patient relationship, neonatal research, appropriate physical liability, and the value of continuing existence in an intensive care unit. In this way, in conjunction with the highly profitable business of heath care, comparatively few resources were spent on prevention, curing curable ailments, resolving conflicts of interest between business and the health care community, or the evaluation of research topics.

I expressed my deep empathy for Dr. Death's hectic schedule, but regardless of my efforts to be amicable, I was absolutely denied an earlier appointment.

I called Dr. Goodbody in desperation. Dr. Goodbody is well known for efficient and effective service. Analogous to three young African-American males walking into a store to shop in Georgetown and expecting to be graciously received as potential customers but instead being received as probable thieves, it was not outside the sphere of possibility to expect death from Dr. Goodbody. But the receptionist who took and quickly evaluated my preappointment information, advised me, that the services of the good doctor, so well known for saving lives, would first require extensive tests. I simply left my name and telephone number, requesting that I be advised of the good doctor's next opening for an examination, prior to tests.

In truth, the receptionist did not actually tell me that I could not see or afford Dr. Goodbody's services. Rather, this conclusion was based on common sense and *The American Journal of Medicine*, which establishes correlations between whether a person has private insurance, Medicaid, or no insurance and the type of treatment he or she receives. Being black in a racist society, I thought, could only aggravate the likelihood of maltreatment. I have private insurance and an HMO, so why should I give Dr. Goodbody a blank check to perform unneeded services and face the prospects of receiving from the same Dr. Goodbody a less than adequate diagnosis? Although I wanted the results of Dr. Goodbody's services, namely, death, I did not want to be exploited in the process.

Refusing to dethrone my honor by calling in sick, having the option of seeing Dr. Death foreclosed, and even my most readily available institutionalized source for death, Dr. Goodbody, excluded from my short list of possible harm providers, I resolved to live with my apprehension as fait accompli. Moreover, I counted myself fortunate because my apprehension was not a pancreatic cancer.

This unusual way of constructing honor and the drastic effort to avoid completing and presenting my paper may seem unreasonable, particularly because other options were available. I could have written the Center, explained my apprehension, and refused to submit my paper or to present it. I could have elected to go on a holiday with no thought of Dr. Death or an unfinished paper. I could have re-evaluated the situation in the light of the fact that I really could not predict how my paper would be received. I could have completed my paper, but submitted it for publication to a reputable journal and if it were published, I would improve my chances for promotion in academia and simultaneously avoid the probability of needing to defend my views. I could have sought psychiatric help to overcome my apprehension, discovered its root or contributing factors, and acquired a greater sense of self-confidence—regardless of whether greater confidence, rather than less apprehension, would enhance my psychological stability.

What's rational requires taking into account variables that are not immediately on the surface of initial considerations. It is no small matter, for example, to have respondents from Georgetown University and Harvard University—particularly so as I am a professor at a small historically black college, a philosopher in an era when philosophy has nearly lost its status, a radical author, and an African-American promoting the idea of struggle against authority. The following were a few hidden concerns: Will I be perceived as representing the quality of professors at Morgan? Will I be perceived as representing all African-Americans? Will my project of promoting the history and heritage of African-American philosophic activity fare well before such distinguished respondents? Will they find my revaluations of the bioethical agenda totally afield of the way biomedical ethics is now constituted and in the future reject efforts by others to raise the same issues without due consideration because they were prejudiced by a poor paper from me? If my views are not defensible, will it be inferred that I am genetically inferior or defective? These questions and the meanings they convey dictate the fact that it is no small matter to have two distinguished respondents.

Taking hidden variables into account enriches but cannot dictate the outcome of considerations. What type of deference I am accorded, how important my presence is in the world, how significant my problem is to the corporate body of society, and what type of autonomy I am assumed to possess, are affected by what kind of rational agent I am considered to be. Considering my apprehension a substantive matter, and the above options drastic but not insane, for example, accords me regard as a reasoning agent, if not a rational agent. That is, outside the context of what presenting and presenting with two distinguished respondents means in a racist world, my reasoning arguably does not warrant regarding me as a rational agent. Instead it warrants considering me less than fully rational because it is full of over-generalizations and fallacies—precisely the kind of reasoning characteristic of actual well and poorly-educated persons.[5]

THE BODY AS SOCIALLY ENWEBBED

My peculiar original reasoning, whether considered rational, misguided, or just peculiar does not affect perceiving me as an autonomous agent per se. The good that I have as an autonomous agent, however, is encased in a context that affects how beneficial my autonomy is to me. It is a dubious good, for example, in a social world in which my miseries are considered my responsibility in at least two senses: if they were preventable, then my choice-making activities were a major factor; if not preventable, then what is to be done is a function of my choices under duress. A functional argument can be made contending that the concept of autonomy readily allows health care professionals to blame victims, render less than adequate services, or withhold cures. To the extent that autonomy excuses society and health care professionals from responsibility and accountability to initiate life practices to prevent ailment, the benefit of being perceived as autonomous also carries harm. I do not, however, wish to offer a functional argument here.

The "body-as-object" is not, I believe, a physical phenomenon strictly separate from how it is socially constructed—and its construction involves relying on beliefs about the agent's rational being.[6] Assuming I gain entrance to Dr. Death, for example, the diagnosis and prognosis are affected by the status of my body in a web of beliefs about its merit. Whether, for example, I am constructed as "inferior, irrational, or hyperactive" prior to or independent of test results stands along side concerns such as "Can I really afford the services or am I really a social pariah usurping taxpayer funds?" Assuming that I am accidentally, or because of moral luck, treated by a decent physician, that I am treated at all is conditioned by social factors and not the sheer objective existence of a physical ailment. Whether autonomy is considered an end state or an existential process of becoming; whether authenticity or a principle of bodily integrity and respect is considered of greater importance, the status of the agent affects their application. Autonomy, consequently, can be a dubious good for persons socially constructed as inferior.

The concept of the body as socially enwebbed may be controversial, and it is a concept that phenomenologists have argued for in far more detail than I will attempt. I rely on a weak form of the idea: that "objective" physical reality is necessarily mediated by subjective meanings. This view is fairly noncontroversial. However, when considered in connection to how the immiserated are treated, the idea suggests a departure from conceiving of the body as an object such that appropriate health care entails proper application of technology mediated by rational physicians. That is, a physical ailment would not simply be an object for pure science or medicine to observe, but an object embedded in a myriad of perspectives that intrinsically and extrinsically encode it with meaning. Hypertension, diabetes, and AIDS, for example, are among the most common ailments afflicting the African-American community (as if these conditions were ailments emanating from outside agents). If not totally preventable, at least the number of persons affected by these conditions could be reduced by alterations in social life. But to treat the social as the prime source of affliction (again, as if the ailments emanated from outside agents), is to conceive of the body in a social and phenomenological fashion (as a dialectical entwinement of object and subject).

What health is should be considered as an extension of a conception of the subject, i.e., how the subject's being is to be perceived. Conceptions such as "autonomy" presuppose the existence of an essentially common humanity. How humanity is constructed is thus crucial to a defensible view of autonomy. Species membership, I believe, is adequate for encoding an undifferentiated quintessence of personhood to species' members. How functional, utilitarian, or capable we are of empathy with a given member of the species in actual or imagined contractual relations should be separate issues from whether agents are accorded peership as human persons.

CHALLENGING THE EPISTEME

It is arguable that if we have a sufficiently rich rule-governed conception of autonomy, well founded in ethical principles such that the autonomy of agents is given due respect, we should be able to apply conceptions and principles in ways that help limit socially demeaning characterizations of persons. An appropriate application would, as a consequence of a diagnostic reasoning procedure, render fair applications. It can be argued consequently that we could, with appropriate corrective procedures, require consideration of persons with equal regard as species' members.

Contrary to the Platonic ideal, injustice often pays because the unjust do not act alone but in a community that sanctions and makes injustice normal, restricting "greatest injustice to barbarians and outlanders."[7] Moreover, an intrinsically good person is not necessarily inclined either to know or to do good acts, particularly under duress. An absolutely congruent fit between principles and their application, such that the principle and an accompanying procedure necessarily tell us incontrovertibly what to do in all relevant cases, is not possible. Noting the impossibility of an absolute congruent fit between principles, procedures, and actions, I believe, is not controversial, but the recognition that the best possible fit could be foreshadowed by how the "other" is constructed suggests the need for considerations besides rule-governed procedures and correctives. The idea I am arguing for is that a conception of rule-governed principles constituting one singular rule or a lexical arrangement of rules from which we can inductively generate right actions is inadequate. Principles and practices, whether derived by uninterested rational agents or whether they are as justifiable as we can make them, do not escape the need for the existence of a critical standpoint toward social reality, i.e., a critique that attacks how objects are categorized, constructed, constituted, and encoded with meaning.

It is not unusual for persons to arrange hierarchically the valuation of nonmoral goods. Societies, for example, characteristically value wealth, income, status, type of profession, power, and material possessions. The ill, poor, unemployed, and powerless are usually not as valued as persons with health, wealth, and power. Hauserman remarks that, "the essence of the problem lies in the transference of such characteristic values to consideration of the human being as a whole. Society infers that the values associated with an individual's biological differences are indicative of the individual's overall personal values."[8] The sort of respect, deference, accord, regard, attention and autonomy a person is assumed to warrant, at least in informal considerations, is affected by and affects, the biological standing of persons. Background assumptions that shape how the body is formally or informally categorized constitute its meaning for the physician. Consequently, although a given physician may believe in a rule-governed principle of autonomy, and apply its rules judiciously, a sphere that configures prejudicial and demeaning practices may be left unaffected.

The primary markers determining a person's access to health care and their rank are social constructions, e.g., class, race, religion, clan, nationality, or material accoutrements. They exist prior to a person's treatment by a physician. They effect how a person is ranked. Which markers are used depends on the society. Moreover, the traits of rationality, autonomy, independence, or authenticity are imputed in the sense that third parties are required to confirm, verify, grant, or award individuals such goods; and on confirmation, determine what may or may not be done under normal conditions or conditions of duress. Whether, and in what form, an individual has such traits may be legitimately controversial; however, that persons are entitled to recognition as persons is not, and due regard should not, in an ideal world, be a matter of third party evaluations.

Given the tendency to transfer valuations of nonmoral goods to valuations of persons, and assuming the continued existence of social markers, how subjects are primordially constituted is crucial to the possibility of equitable health care—the possibility of a health care system that is not complicit in immiseration. The minimally adequate level of autonomy that should be accorded persons across lines of social differentiation requires a conception of the subject that grants agents intrinsic good independent of and prior to ranking or countervailing considerations. A conception is needed that constructs agents as undifferentiated.

It is not, consequently, that the "principles to practice" mode of constructing reasoning is psychologically a mode of thinking that does not occur, or one that we should abandon, but that there are background assumptions and intervening considerations that procedural ethical reasoning cannot take into account because background assumptions surreptitiously legitimate or call into question procedures and the context of procedures. By calling the context of procedures into question I mean revaluation of what is meant by normalcy, authenticity, respect and independence.

Historically, African-Americans and persons focused on ending the immiseration of blacks have forced the positive consciousness of knowledge, its epistemological figures, its taken-for-grantedness, its "too-obviously-true-to-warrant-critiqueness," its philosophy of life, into and onto the social, intellectual, literary, and medical state for critique.[9] We should certainly clarify principles, struggle for an invigorating ethos, and promote a covenant that inspires community. We should also continue to struggle over which conception of health, ethos, covenants and methodological applications are defensible. The point is that this intellectual and practical struggle occurs on a background that must itself be continually revaluated and that the struggle includes how the subject is to be constituted.

The critiques offered by African-Americans, acting from various perspectives and as agents of resistance, reshape the subject and challenge the *episteme* on which the health care system grounds itself. Contrary to the ideal of an all-seeing eye peering down on a static biological world of homo sapiens awaiting discovery of their finite and predefined categories, African-American critiques often tender a critical judgment about the *episteme*, the intervening background assumptions and socially constituted configuration of subjects that precondition the object and the eye.

An arguable implication of this view is that a good deal more than promoting humanitarian beliefs and antiprejudicial attitudes is required to abate racism. The reason for this is that physicians are not understood as simply subjective agents peering out, hopefully through the spectrum of rational thinking, at an objective body. Rather, the body is a socially constructed and constituted subject entwined and configured by the physician and the physician's social context. If race-targeted advertising such as cigarette and alcohol advertising elicit less social consternation than we might hope, one reason may be that the target is not invested by physicians and society in general with ties of affection, compassion, kinship, merit, and value among those empowered to create change. This may be true whether those empowered are African-Americans, reluctant to vie against their fellow health care professionals or whites, invested with a sense of class, but not race, superiority.

If we are not sufficiently aggressive in instituting cultural change to influence dietary habits as a way of curtailing diabetes, one reason may be that Africans and African-Americans shy away from being thoroughly self-critical since they are already subject to so many demeaning criticisms. Offering our own critique may seem only to add to the harm. Or empowered health care professionals may feel that authenticity demands allowing the least well off to immiserate themselves as a function of their independence (that is, they are constituted as independent agents just in case self-immiseration occurs, or they are constituted as full persons deserving counseling just in case their actions or presence seriously influence others constituted as full persons). Moreover, what are considered public health matters of great importance, such as infant mortality or drug-addicted pregnant women, reflect the status of worth accorded different sectors of the population. Consequently, how we constitute the subject, as intrinsically worthy anterior to experience and due intransitive regard, are important grounds from which to fight racism.

I have not offered a sufficient view of health or the health care system, nor have I depicted a unique African-American perspective on health or the role of healers and patients in the African or African-American culture. There are certainly folk, religious, historical, and culturally popular beliefs about health among African people. There are certainly numerous African-based continuities helping to shape those beliefs. Moreover, the African-American experience of the health care system is too often a demeaning experience, and this, on the background of centuries of suspicion. I have not covered the historical details that have informed suspicions that may, for example, account for the small number of black organ donors, attitudes toward advice concerning sexual practices emanating from the health care system, or our reluctance to address race or ethnic-specific treatments, diseases, or cures.

The critical perspective I have presented may include features integral to the array of ways African-American, and African people in general, view health and some concerns regarding patient-physician (as distinct from healer) relations. If it turns out, however, after a searching historical and sociological study of African-American beliefs, that my critical perspective or the importance I place on the resistance tradition among African-American health care professionals is not integral to that perspective—then it should be. Moreover, if an African-American perspective does not exist, I would argue that there are strong grounds for creating one in the history and continued immiseration of African people by health care systems.

(I have completed my paper. I am now worried that Dr. Goodbody will actually see—and therefore construct—me).

NOTES

1. For the import of autonomy and authenticity, some examples include: Gerald Dworkin, "Moral Autonomy," in *Morals, Sciences and Sociality*, vol. 3 of *The Foundations of Ethics and Its Relationship to Science*, ed. H. Tristram Engelhardt, Jr., and Daniel Callahan (New York: The Hastings Center, 1978); "Autonomy and Behavior Control," *Hastings Center Report* (February 1976) 6:23; Bruce Miller, "Autonomy and the Refusal of Life-Saving Treatment," *Hastings Center Report* (August 1981) 11:22-28.

For the import of autonomy and self-respect, some examples include James Childress, *Who Should Decide?: Paternalism in Health Care* (Oxford: Oxford University Press, 1982); John Rawls, *A Theory of Justice* (Massachusetts: Harvard University Press, 1971); Robert Nozick, *Anarchy, State, and Utopia* (New York: Basic Books, 1974), 28-35.

2. For the rituals of lynching and justifications of lynching and castration, see Trudier Harris, *Exorcising Blackness*, (Bloomington, Indiana: Indiana University Press, 1984); and Robert L. Zangrando, *The NAACP Crusade Against Lynching* (Philadelphia: Temple University Press, 1980).

3. For the concept of natal alienation, see Orlando Patterson, *Slavery and Social Death* (Massachusetts: Harvard University Press, 1982).

4. Nancy R. Hauserman, "Search for Equity on the Planet Difference" in *Biological Differences and Social Equality*, ed. Masako N. Darrough and Robert H. Blank (Westport, Connecticut: Greenwood Press, 1983), 27.

5. For the concept of epistemological figures and *episteme*, see Michel Foucault, *The Order of Things: An Archaeology of the Human Sciences* (New York, Random House, 1970).

For the concept of valuation and the integral way values help shape cultural imports, see Alain Locke, "Values and Imperatives" in Leonard Harris, *The Philosophy of Alain Locke* (Philadelphia: Temple University Press, 1989).

6. See Michel Feher, et.al., *Fragments for a History of the Body*, I, II, Urzone, 1989.

7. Boxill, Bernard, "How Injustice Pays," *Philosophy & Public Affairs*, 9:4 (Summer 1980): 369.

8. Nancy R. Hauserman, "Search for Equity on the Planet Difference," in *Biological Differences and Social Equality*, ed. Masako N. Darrough and Robert H. Blank (Westport, Connecticut: Greenwood Press, 1983), 27.

9. For the concept of epistemological figures and *episteme*, see note 5; for the concept of valuation and the integral way values help shape cultural imports, see Alain Locke, "Values and Imperatives," in Leonard Harris, *The Philosophy of Alain Locke,* (Philadelphia: Temple University Press, 1989).

Edmund D. Pellegrino:

Response to Leonard Harris

Professor Harris's "Poplar Tree Narrative" is a perceptive, poignant, and pungent critique of the dominant mode of doing ethics. Though his critique is shaped by his African-American perspective, its significance transcends culture. It underscores the difficulties inherent in any culturally shaped ethic. His discussion is pertinent, therefore, for all of ethics, biomedical or general.

Clearly Harris's paper has implications beyond those I can explore in a short commentary. I will confine myself to what I conceive to be the major point in Harris's thesis, namely, that the dominant theories of ethics and the principles that we espouse are shaped by deeper, often unexpressed cultural presuppositions. As a consequence, principle-based ethics and moral judgments based on deductive reasoning from principles are necessary but not sufficient foundations for a valid moral philosophy. To understand and criticize any ethical system we must lay bare its presuppositions. I would only add that once cultural presuppositions have been explicated, they too must be subject to critical examination.

Thus, while I am in agreement with Professor Harris's critique of current ethical discourse and justification I would like to carry it further. Granting that the character of moral reasoning, principles, and judgments is determined by cultural presuppositions, how do we judge among cultures? Are they self-justifying? Are there morally good and morally evil cultures or parts of cultures? Is it enough to understand how culture shapes ethics? Does not the fact that culture so profoundly shapes ethics require a metacultural foundation by which cultures themselves may be judged?

Harris makes two assertions. First, that "there are background assumptions and intervening considerations that procedural ethical reasoning cannot take into account because background assumptions surreptitiously legitimate or call into question procedures and the context of procedures."[1] Second, and precisely because of the first, we always have need of "a critique that attacks how objects are categorized, constituted, and encoded with meaning."[2] I agree with both these assumptions. I wish Professor Harris had followed up on the second point, however, because without it his critique loses normative force. The culture that gave birth to Dr. Dick's distorted moral judgments cannot be judged invalid without some criteria outside that culture against which its moral quality can be measured. This is a logical extrapolation of Harris's major thesis, and I wish to examine it further in this commentary.

In the "Poplar Tree Narrative" Dr. Dick, a conscientious physician, applies the prima facie principles of beneficence, autonomy, and justice in such a way that castration of his black male patient is construed as a morally justifiable act, in substance and as a procedure. In Dick's view, mutilation of a black male slave's body keeps that male, in this case George Washington Carver, from getting into "trouble." As a result he is prevented from falling into compromising and dangerous "situations" with white females. As a eunuch he can be a better slave, a more productive member of the household, and lead a happier, more peaceful life. Society will be well served.

Dick even "protects" Carver's autonomy by getting what he construes to be Carver's informed consent. Harris thus shows how Dr. Dick's cultural presuppositions constitute Carver's body, Carver's good, and the good of black people and society as a whole. Harris shows that given his presuppositions, Dr. Dick's conclusions can be deduced on either consequentialist or deontological grounds. Those presuppositions are also powerful in defining Dr. Dick's conception of illness and health and his relationship as physician to his patient.

Harris shows clearly that prima facie principles do not stand alone. They are embedded in a cultural matrix that encodes them with meaning. Carver and his body were so constituted by the Southern slave culture that autonomy for him was a travesty. For a black male in that culture, autonomy was simply functionally nonexistent. Similarly, maleficence became beneficence and injustice became justice. Dr. Dick's deduction of the right and good from these principles was logical but faulted because his background assumptions were morally wrong.

But how can we say that Dr. Dick's culture was wrong? We beg the fundamental question if we cannot point to some criteria by which we condemn the cultural presuppositions that legitimized Dr. Dick's actions. Is every culture self-justifying? Is there any way to discriminate between a good and a bad culture without using one culture to arbitrarily criticize another? Is there a moral reality more fundamental than culture? Must we be content with an infinite relativity of moral values, each with an equal claim to truth? Or, is there a source of normative values that is not relative to the culture in which such values reside? Professor Harris does not address these questions. They go beyond the descriptive definition of culture customary to anthropology and the social sciences. They require a philosophy of culture.

The social sciences have enriched our knowledge with details of a wide spectrum of cultures and within cultures. These details are essential starting points for any critical inquiry into the moral quality of cultures. The purpose of a philosophy of culture is not, arbitrarily, to select one culture—Western, Eastern, or African—as the standard to which the others must conform. Rather, it asks, from the point of view of our common humanity, what are the characteristics of a morally defensible culture?[3] If there is no answer to this question, or none is deemed possible, then there is no foundation for judging the presuppositions of Dr. Dick's ethics to be morally distorted. Such a conclusion, except for the skeptic, is patently unacceptable. Therefore, difficult as it may be, some criteria beyond culture must be sought by which any cultures may be judged.

Before examining the sources for such criteria, it is necessary to define the sense in which I am using the word "culture." The word "culture" has many shades of meaning, anthropological, sociological, and philosophical. Culture is a product of humankind but also, once established, it is a shaper of humanity.[4] It may be taken broadly to embrace all of humanity or more narrowly it may be confined to individual cultures. The interactions between individuals and their culture are exceedingly complex. Their many nuances are beyond the competence or scope of this commentary. Nonetheless it is essential, if one is to speak at all of "culture," to provide at least an operational definition. I take culture to be the sum total of the ways a people respond to the several worlds in which we live as humans—the inner world of self, the outer worlds of others, of nature, and the transcendental. Humans, because they are endowed with intelligence, feelings, and a social nature, express their responses to these realities in language, thought, emotion, art, myth, religion, and social organization. A group that shares the same set of responses constitutes a "culture." That culture is a group's "world view," a selection of values and priorities about that which has meaning and importance for it.

Culture in this sense has positive and negative features. On the positive side, culture provides group and self-identity, support against alien intruders, stability, continuity, and a shared way of life, social communication, support, and moral guidelines. Culture thus enriches and fulfills, but it also controls and limits the life we lead. It enjoins certain kinds of behavior and prohibits others. To be part of a culture is to incur duties of fidelity to the values that identify the culture. Not to respect cultural values is to be a pariah.

These strengths of cultural identity are also its weaknesses. By identifying with one set of values and not another, cultures become exclusive. Those who have different values and duties are aliens, threatening, and somehow not quite fully human. The Greeks for example saw anyone who did not speak the Greek language as a "barbarian" (βαρβαρος).[5]

The way Dr. Dick constituted the body and person of George Washington Carver made Carver something less than human. For the Nazis, the Jews and all non-Aryans were outside the human pale. For the Soviet psychiatrists, political dissidents were mentally incapacitated. For the Latin American physicians who tortured their political prisoners, these prisoners had no human rights. Similarly, Christians and Moslems for centuries have labelled each other "infidels", i.e., those "without faith" in the "true" values. Cultures are supportive for those who share their moral vision, divisive for those who do not. How far is it possible to go in respecting cultural differences without balkanizing segments of a society? Can our differences be our contributions to each other? Or will they prove so irreconcilable as to be socially disruptive?

These tensions are particularly urgent in practical biomedical ethics because so many of its relationships are based on inequalities of power and vulnerability. Today, the probabilities are high that physicians and patients will not share the same culture. Yet, they must interact in matters of life and death just at those points at which different cultures are most likely to be in conflict. The "melting pot" concept is no longer a panacea for cultural diversity. Many minorities see it not as a way of unifying the nation but of subverting non-European values and cultures.

In what direction may one turn for a common ground for societal intercourse and ethical judgment? Ultimately, it must be some foundation even more elemental than culture. What must be faced in Professor Harris's challenge is that there is no way to mount a rational argument against the immorality of Dr. Dick's culture other than to appeal to some metacultural moral foundation beyond cultural bias.

We need not, at this point, argue whether such a metacultural foundation is best based on some logical Archimedean starting point or some emotionally felt universal sentiment. Is there, as both Professors Banner and Harris have asked, something more decisive for ethics than culture?[6] Is there something common to all human experience that can reliably judge the ethical quality of cultures? Some would immediately say no. We have only the history, culture, and myths by which people live. To seek something prior is an illusion that can lead to outmoded naturalism or overly presumptuous a priorism. On this view, we would have to be satisfied with the radical relativism both of standards and judgments (to use Tom Beauchamp's distinction).[7] There would be no way to criticize Dr. Dick's cultural distortion of ethics. By what right could anyone challenge Dr. Dick, if culture were self-justifying? The only resource would be some negotiated compromise or consensus on cultural values. But this becomes more difficult the more it engages the fundamental questions of philosophical anthropology: what is a human person? What is owed to each of us as persons?

Those for whom radical, cultural, and ethical relativism is unacceptable, have two philosophical recourses: a philosophy of human nature and a philosophy of medicine, both of which must be grounded in human realities that transcend cultural differences in essential ways. For while cultures differ, they are all the products of human ingenuity, of something peculiar to humans that does not exist in other species.

What is the source of this peculiar characteristic of the human species that gives rise to culture but also transcends it? Aristotle asked and answered this question as well as it can be answered: "but we are asking," he says, "what is peculiar to man."[8] After eliminating nutrition, growth, and sensation as activities that other species share with humankind, Aristotle concludes that "There remains then, an active life of the element that has a rational principle . . . and we state the function of man to be a certain kind of life and this to be an activity or actions of the soul implying rational principle and the function of a good man to be the good and noble performance of these."[9]

This quality of leading the active life of a being that has reason is common to all humans whatever culture they belong to. It is this quality that makes the formation of a culture possible in the first place and provides the possibility of judging the activity of culture-making, i.e., whether or not the "the performance" is good and noble.

All of us share this capability for rationality. We also all have feelings and emotions. We worry, suffer, die, have intimate relationships with others, share certain basic needs and seek happiness and per-

sonal fulfillment. We plan, hope, aspire, succeed, and fail. We become
ill, go through the stages of life, and die. We are capable of moral
agency, possess consciences, and seek the good. We live with consciousness of a past, anticipate the future, and elaborate cultures.

Taken together these are features distinctive of humanity, and the
foundation of the moral claims humans have on each other as humans. To respect the equality of every human's claim to the operation
of one's full humanity, certain obligations are binding on all; that is,
we are not to harm but help each other, not to usurp but enhance
each other's freedom, to render to each what is owed and to recognize the claims of others as limits on our own autonomy.

These moral claims are based in our common human nature.
They provide the metacultural basis of ethics and the criteria for a critique of the ethical presuppositions of a culture. Violations or distortions of these claims are the marks of an ethically faulted culture.
Only from the vantage point of the moral claims of humans qua humans can a rational critique be made of the distorted ethical perspective that made the mutilation of George Washington Carver a
heinous act no matter what his doctor or culture may have justified.
Professor Harris's Poplar Tree Narrative has ethical meaning only if
Carver's inherent worth is derived from something beyond his own
or Dr. Dick's cultures.

I appreciate that many would not accept Aristotle's philosophy as
a basis for our common morality. The idea of "human nature" has
been under attack since the writings of the British empiricist philosophers of the eighteenth century. Some may also reject the Aristotelian
view as only partially adequate since it neglects humanity's spiritual
telos. I subscribe to this view, but have limited myself to the minimum requirements in attempts to come closer to some possibility of
agreement. In any case, the major point here is that without some
foundation for ethics in a philosophical anthropology, the kinds of
cultural presuppositions Professor Harris rightly condemns are difficult to refute.

If we turn to a more restricted and more immediate arena of ethical discourse, biomedical ethics, there may be more hope for agreement. The telos of medicine is narrower than the telos of humanity
qua humanity. Within a phenomenologically based ethics of the healing relationship, I believe we can find a metacultural basis for a critique of professional ethics.

In the more narrow confines of the physician-patient relationship,
the healing relationship, there are also ethical claims that transcend
culture. To be sure, medicine and professional ethics exist in a cultural context. Their principles and rules are shaped, like those of

ethics in general, by cultural presuppositions as the Poplar Tree Narrative shows. But the ethics of medicine is also derived from an experience and a set of relationships that are peculiar to medicine as a certain kind of human activity, common to humans as humans and therefore beyond any particular culture. In fact we have a set of obligations intrinsic to medicine as an activity that would have imposed on Dr. Dick the moral necessity of standing against the presuppositions of his culture.

Some might immediately object and point out that health, illness, modes of healing, and medicine are inextricably culture bound. Are not theories of medicine defined in cultural terms? Would I not be using the ethical precepts of modern western medicine and committing the sin of Eurocentrism?

I think not. What I propose is something more fundamental than a cultural theory of medicine. I refer to the common human experience of illness—the universal experience of pain, anxiety, dependance, vulnerability, suffering, the sense of alienation from the world of the well, and having to meet the emotional and spiritual challenge to the self of being forced to trust in those who care for us. However one defines illness and disease—ontologically, nominalistically, or socio-culturally, the human experience of illness has certain common characteristics.[10] That is, a human in distress is in need of the help of another who offers himself as a healer—a neurosurgeon or a shaman. The vulnerable state of the sick person and one's need for help, and the inequality in power between the patient and healer—all these phenomena impose obligations on the healer. These obligations derive from moral claims—e.g., obligations to act in the best interest of the sick person, to accord him or her all the moral rights we have defined above for any human being, and to pay special attention to his or her vulnerable and exploitable state. Taken together these obligations make up that part of medical ethics that goes beyond culture. It is these phenomena that give meaning to principles like beneficence, justice and autonomy, and the derived principles of truth-telling, promise-keeping, and confidentiality. These obligations are binding no matter what a culture may do to distort them. They constitute the metacultural criteria for morally valid healing. Dr. Dick and the Nazi doctors violated them. No argument based on cultural uniqueness or difference can excuse their offense against the ethics of healing.

It is reassuring on this point and to medicine's credit, that those common obligations have been recognized in the professional codes of different cultures, e.g., the Greek, Roman, Indian, Jewish, and Chinese codes.[11] While each code is embedded in a different cultural and historical era, each promulgates essentially the same obligations.

Physicians in every culture have dared to speak up and to stand for the sick against the culture itself.

Clearly, we cannot justify a plurality of medical ethical systems each based in special cultural presuppositions. There is only one set of morally defensible principles and duties owed sick persons. Even the existence of past prejudice and injustice do not justify ethical systems that violate the basic moral claims of the sick and the moral obligations of the doctor. Indeed, the only way to prevent the injustice perpetrated on George Washington Carver in the Poplar Tree Narrative is to discern precisely at what point cultural presuppositions transgress the morality inherent in the healing relationship. None of this precludes taking into account the history of a race, the restitution of past injustice, the reality of ethnic and culture differences, and differences in response to illness. Indeed, a valid medical ethic, based in the phenomenon of illness and healing would respect and encompass those differences, while a culturally limited medical ethic might not feel itself obligated to do so.

Professor Harris's Poplar Tree Narrative made a convincing case for intercultural dialogue of the kind we are having at this conference. In that dialogue we must recognize and respect the values of cultural differences, but we must also seek out the metacultural sources of ethics. We need well grounded criteria for judgment when cultural presuppositions distort the obligations we owe to each other as humans and to all sick persons as humans. We need to work toward a common philosophy of humanity, and of medicine as the ground of ethics. The task is formidable. But the alternative is, as Professor Harris has so eloquently observed, the possibility of falsely constituting, the body, mind, and spirit of those outside our own culture.

Culture, like government, can be the source of fulfillment or of tyranny. Eventually, we must work toward some world culture based on what it is to be human, and what it is to be sick. This larger culture should be broad enough to encompass the strengths of cultural diversity and strong enough to prevent the subjugation of ethics by the more limited and circumscribed perspectives of particular cultures. Given the ubiquity of cultural, nationalist, and religious strife in today's world, the hope of recognizing something beyond cultural parochialism seems remote. But if the George Washington Carvers of our world are ever to be safe from cultural exploitation and injustice, we must not abandon the effort.

NOTES

1. Leonard Harris, "Autonomy under Duress," in this volume.

2. Ibid.

3. Donald P. Verene *Man and Culture* (New York: Dell, 1970), 4-6; Ernst Cassirer *An Essay on Man* (New York: Bantam Pub. Co., 1970), 252.

4. Miecyzlaw A. Krapiec, *I-Man: An Outline of Philosophical Anthropology* (New Britain: Mariel Publications, 1983), 170-171; Francisco Romero, *Theory of Man* (Berkeley: University of California Press, 1964), 117-118, 96-97.

5. Cf. *Iliad* 2.867 and Stabo, *Geographicus* 14.2.

6. Leonard Harris, "Autonomy under Duress" (in this volume), and William Banner, "Response to Jorge Garcia" (in this volume).

7. Tom Beauchamp, "Response to Jorge Garcia," in this volume.

8. Aristotle, *Nichomachean Ethics*, in *The Basic Works of Aristotle*, trans. W. D.Ross (New York: Pantheon Press, 1973), 1097b, 34.

9. Ibid., 1098a, 2-3; 11-14.

10. Arthur L. Caplan, H. Tristram Engelhardt, and James J. McCarney (ed.), *Concepts of Health and Disease, Interdisciplinary Perspectives* (Massachusetts: Addison Wesley Press, 1981).

11. See, for example, Ludwig Edelstein's "The Hippocratic Oath," *Ancient Medicine*, ed. Owsei Temkin (Baltimore: Johns Hopkins University Press, 1967), 3-64; R. Walzer's "New Light on Galen's Moral Philosophy," in *Oriental Studies I* (1962); *Galen's* On Natural Faculties, trans. A. J. Brock (Cambridge: Harvard University Press, 1957).

Lynn M. Peterson:

Response to Leonard Harris

Professor Harris describes some unsatisfactory medical care events. What do these descriptions mean? Should or can anything be done to improve health care for the African-American? My comments will reflect the point of view of a practicing surgeon and Director of a Division of Medical Ethics. Professor Harris's criticism and struggle must be taken seriously. He identifies real problems in trying to move from principles to practices. These problems can be aided by a better understanding of the background assumptions, subtexts, and webs of meaning that Dr. Harris identifies. He is correct that autonomy is not the bottom line, though it is one component in the moral argument and deserves the attention of scholars and health care providers.

The healers or the health care system in Professor Harris's three examples made mistakes. Recognizing these events as mistakes rather than accidents or misfortunes is an important first step in defining the problems at hand. Once we have defined a problem, then we can start thinking about its correction. In part, Dr. Harris challenges us to provide a more patient-centered style of care.

My remarks examine three issues raised in Dr. Harris's paper: (1) The conflicting roles and responsibilities of health care providers and how these conflicts were causally related to the mistakes; (2) When and how the African-American perspective should make a difference in the health care setting; and (3) What we can learn and teach if we take the first two items seriously.

CONFLICTING ROLES

Yesterday Professor Wiredu presented the Akan view of the person or moral agent as the center of a series of concentric circles or relations, responsibilities, and rights. Professor Hehir then recognized a convergence between this Akan image and the Catholic notion that a person has different levels of responsibility. Both views demonstrate, therefore, that people are innately social beings, having multiple responsibilities and interests.

Recognizing layers, circles, or levels of responsibility, however, is only part of the problem. Fulfilling these multiple levels of responsibility is a major challenge. The potential for conflict is enormous. Conflicts may occur within a role; physicians, for example, have duties to be loyal to their colleagues and to report fraud and deception. Conflicts may occur between roles; a nurse who finds abortion morally wrong may not be able to fulfill her nursing duties during an abortion. Finally, conflicts may be temporal; it may be impossible to see patients in the emergency room while at the same time seeing patients with scheduled office visits.

One way to deal with these conflicts is to describe an ideal behavior—a gold standard—for a particular role, then set priorities in reference to that ideal. This at least enables one to be explicit with others in reference to that ideal. Letting others know what they can expect may promote their comfort. More important it establishes coherence between one's basic, most fundamental, moral beliefs and one's personal or professional actions.

Parenthetically we may note that technology not only makes it possible to keep people alive longer but also changes the role responsibilities of doctors, nurses, physician assistants, and others. One person can no longer know or do everything for a particular patient. Complex technology increasingly creates the need for shared and shifting responsibilities—and new possibilities for conflict.

Professor Harris describes three doctors who perform in such a way that their actions fail to fulfill what we would ordinarily consider the professional ideal, i.e., either a procedure was wrongfully done, or access to care was denied. An "ideal" doctor should act in a way that promotes the patient's interests, respects the patient's autonomy, avoids unnecessary harm, uses medical resources prudently, and avoids wasteful practices. Let's look at Professor Harris's cases to see what went wrong.

First, Dr. Dick castrates George Washington Carver. In that example Dr. Dick carries out a purely social policy. He alters a slave to suit the needs of a master. Second, he does so in the belief that he is preventing the possibility of an even more egregious injustice—the lynching of an African-American suspected of rape. In so doing, however, Dr. Dick was not fulfilling his central medical duty of helping to heal patients with bonafide medical diseases; he was providing a social service.

Providing such a service may not, in itself, be wrong, but Dr. Dick should have been more careful. Physicians who have been involved in torture and capital punishment have similarly erred. A specific example of such a mistake was the distribution of penicillin by medical doctors in the North African theater in the early phases of World War II. Military physicians apparently used the limited supply of penicillin to treat soldiers who had contracted gonorrhea in the brothels to get them back on the front lines. As a result, soldiers wounded in battle were not given penicillin. The physician's treatment was determined by a strictly social, utilitarian calculus. A better policy from the physician's perspective would have involved a more complex calculus taking into consideration the potential medical benefit (and harm) of the need to have soldiers fit and fighting on the front lines.

In the same fashion, the castration of Dr. Carver was not medically justified. Castration might have been justified for a patient with prostate cancer or testicular cancer but not for social policy objectives. Similar conflicts and errors can occur when doctors are employed by insurance companies or other industries. In these circumstances, the best decision for an individual patient may conflict with what's best for the company.

Dr. Dick's second mistake concerns his belief that a white woman's fetus fertilized by a black man "represented pollution, disease, and corruption." As there is no reason to use the terms "disease" or "infection" in this instance, so there is no medical justification for the abortion.

Services like vasectomy, tubal ligation, abortion, and aesthetic surgery may be justified in many instances. But we need to be clear about these interventions since they are often marginal medical services. As they are primarily designed to help people achieve personal goals, they require that consent be clearly based on realistic expectations and full understanding of the alternatives and risks.

Dr. Death's mistake involved failure to allow timely access for needed care. He apparently took on a number of extra duties in the HMO, making it impossible for him to see a patient with urgent needs. Professor Harris's description shows clearly that doctors are as responsible for access to care as they are for curing and prevention. Several questions arise: (1) Was the HMO understaffed? (2) Did Dr.

Death fail to arrange for someone to cover for him? (3) Was there a system for providing urgent care within the HMO? (4) Was there a failure in communication between the receptionist and the patient?

Dr. Goodbody's mistake involved overly zealous attention to efficiency and exclusion of patients on the basis of ability to pay. Although Principle VI of the American Medical Association's Code of Ethics says a doctor has the "right to choose" the clients he or she will care for, refusing to care on the grounds of inability to pay is totally inconsistent with the doctor's "ideal." This does not mean that doctors are required to ignore fiscal reality; they cannot be expected to make inordinate sacrifices or even jeopardize the existence of their practice. Nevertheless, a doctor should be able to show how refusing to care accomplishes a more important goal.

Dr. Goodbody's second mistake involved unnecessary and possibly wasteful testing. He required tests before the patient even saw a doctor. Had the visit been scheduled first, many of these tests might have been unnecessary.

In summary, we find in Professor Harris's examples three role conflicts: (1) Conflict between the role of the healer versus the role of a provider of social services; (2) The role of the healer versus the role of an HMO employee with some pressure to limit services; and (3) The role of the healer versus the role of an entrepreneur who has an incentive to use more care.

As Dr. Pellegrino has pointed out, these conflicts can be mitigated first by spelling out and then understanding the ideal behavior of health care professionals. Then, efforts must be made to recognize the conflicts and work to minimize them. We need to realize that a moral agent must not only actively pursue the good; he or she must also be prepared to abandon certain roles, e.g., not to provide social services and not always to comply with some institutional or company policies. Only then, will professional agents be especially alert to the difficulties that arise in marginal situations; only then will our actions reiterate the prime importance of the patient's needs and demands.

THE SIGNIFICANCE OF THE
AFRICAN-AMERICAN PERSPECTIVE

Should African-Americans be treated differently? If so, when and how?

The first response, that there should be an equality of care for all people, means indubitably that African-Americans should definitely not receive less care, less attention, or less respect than any other Americans.

In some instances, however, it may be appropriate to consider factors like economic disadvantages, the nature of modern urban life, and a client's lack of adequate social support. When these factors characterize the African-American, as they do other minorities, alterations in the health care process may be justified.

The past history of mistreatment, about which we have heard so much during this conference, appears in background themes of exploitation and immiseration. These factors accentuate anxiety, fear, and disaffection with the health care system, which must therefore make an increased effort to reach out to the community and to be especially patient and sympathetic.

Nurses and doctors frequently represent established authority and are thus seen as threatening or patronizing. We, on the other hand, often consider this authoritarian position as one providing increased confidence and comfort. But illness is a situation in which there is a natural or intrinsic tendency to distrust these power relationships; sometimes they may backfire and breed fear or other adverse reactions. Awareness of this barrier may make it easier to overcome.

The need for family involvement in health care decisions is obvious for people from all cultural backgrounds. Among African-Americans, family involvement may be somewhat different. Aunts, grandmothers, siblings, and children may play different or unexpected roles. Thus, we may need a more careful and different assessment of family connections.

Finally, the existing disparities in health care delivery need to be addressed so that they can be rectified in such a way that African-Americans are not disadvantaged. The most important issue here concerns access. In this regard, health care access needs to be developed in locations and circumstances convenient for African-Americans.

IMPLICATIONS FOR RESEARCH AND TRAINING

What can we do in academic centers to discover and teach optimal practices for caring for African-Americans? Can we improve the health care process?

As Dr. Harris has demonstrated, it seems that enunciating principles of liberty, equality, justice, and respect is only part of the solution. It is the application and interpretation of these principles in complex, concrete situations that need a great deal of attention. We must learn the background factors illustrated in Dr. Harris's talk and how they influence health care delivery before we can act consistently on the basis of these principles.

Part of this learning involves communicating with and understanding individuals from different cultural backgrounds. Words, therefore, are not enough. Attention to nonverbal behavior (for example, facial expressions and gestures) and sensitivity to differences in language use must become part of our research. We can better understand the distress, discomfort, or unhappiness that people experience by broadening our range and sense of communication.

We need to learn how to make subtle distinctions in the interpretation of symptoms and their meaning. Pain, disability, and other kinds of distress may be expressed in a variety of ways.

The use of time is a crucial commodity in professional life. In the case of the African-American, the challenge is to devote enough time to a particular problem. The nontechnical or humane dimension may well require a much greater emphasis.

Finally, Dr. Harris's talk illustrates how existing systems of health care need to be improved. Not only do doctors and nurses need to respond humanely; so do secretaries, laboratory technicians, and clerks. Increasing access and devoting time to the most essential components of care as well as implementing other goals will require more attention to an entire system of care rather than just to isolated individuals or components.

CHERYL J. SANDERS

Problems and Limitations of an African-American Perspective in Biomedical Ethics: A Theological View

In the April 1989 edition of the Kennedy Institute of Ethics *Newsletter*, Harley Flack and Edmund Pellegrino made a preliminary exploration of the importance of African-American perspectives in biomedical ethics. Their brief article reflected on data gathered during a February 1987 conference of African-American scholars, educators, health professionals, and philosophers, and suggested that African-Americans and Anglo-Americans differ in significant ways in their ideas about morality and ethics. They called for further dialogue on the difference in these two cultures in relation to biomedical ethics, the central concern of the present conference.

As a point of departure for my presentation, I would like to focus on a few problematic assertions made in that article, which will help give direction to my own critical analysis of the problems and limitations of an African-American perspective on biomedical ethics. A first problem is Pellegrino and Flack's explanation of the unique nature of the African-American experience as manifested in norms such as the dominant value of community, the importance of religion and an ethics of virtue, and the weight given to personal life experiences:

> Slavery, segregation, discrimination, poverty and a disadvantaged position with respect to education, health and medical care, sensitize African-Americans in specific ways. These experiences evoke a more empathetic response to the social-ethical questions—justice in the distribution of resources, sensitivity to the vulnerability and dependence of the sick person, and a sense of responsibility for the poor and rejected members of society.[1]

165

While their description of the norms of the African-American perspective seems accurate enough, the problem is that they account for this distinctiveness in terms that seriously understate the issue. In their view, the African-American experience is unique because it shows a greater empathy for social-ethical concerns. What they do not say is that the social injustice, insensitivity, and irresponsibility that create this unique state of empathy are direct manifestations of a racist, Anglo-American ethos that is conspicuously indifferent to community, religion, virtue, and personal experience. In other words, it seems absurd to speak of the unique moral context of the African-American experience of suffering without also addressing the cause of this suffering in the broader moral context of Euro-American racism.[2]

A second problem is the call for dialogue and the parenthetical observation that "so few African-Americans are involved in scholarly work in biomedical ethics and how their number might be increased."[3] Again, I take issue not with what is said but with what is left unsaid. Clearly, African-Americans do engage in biomedical ethical discourse on a daily basis, but perhaps not in ways that Euro-Americans regard as scholarly or even noteworthy. Further, it may be that African-Americans have thoughtfully concluded that Western biomedical ethics is not useful or applicable to their dilemmas precisely because their data and input have not been taken into account. In other words, the dialogue being called for may have taken place already in other quarters, and the lack of scholarly work by African-Americans in the field may be indicative of an informed judgment that biomedical ethical discourse is an esoteric and exclusive enterprise in which African-American participation is not really welcome.

Obviously, there is a distinctive African-American ethos that has a direct bearing on biomedical ethics. The real question, then, is not whether such a perspective exists, but why it exists and whether its continued existence is predicated on the persistence of racist oppression of African-American people. Given racism, we must be careful not to fall into the trap of discussing uniqueness rather than universals, so that the African-American perspective becomes strictly valued on the grounds of its uniqueness and not fully appreciated for its universal significance as a critique of the destructive inhumanity of the dominant ethos. Authentic dialogue begins in my opinion when we realize that both perspectives operate within one moral universe not two, and that each brings a valid critique to bear on the other. Both must be subjected to scrutiny by similar standards—it is as erroneous to romanticize African-American culture as it is to overlook the racism that is endemic to Euro-American culture. The point is not that the African-American ethos is unique, but that it is characteristically human in ways that the Euro-American ethos is not. I will discuss the problems and limitations of an African-American perspective in biomedical ethics with reference to the distinctive ethos, theology, and ethics of the African-American people, with a view toward understanding how honest dialogue among African-Americans and Euro-Americans can move us all toward a biomedical ethics that is truly ethical.

THE AFRICAN-AMERICAN ETHOS

Flack and Pellegrino have offered a credible report of the dominant ideas in the African-American perspectives on morals, specifically the greater importance ascribed to community, religion, and the ethics of virtue and personal life experiences in the African-American perspective in comparison to Western value systems. I would like, however, to offer an expanded list of features, seven in all, that describe the African-American ethos or lifestyle, and the corresponding opposites that characterize the Euro-American ethos.

First, the African-American ethos is holistic and nondualistic, emphasizing that most matters are better understood in terms of "both-and" rather than "either-or." Second, it is inclusive, not exclusive, accepting of difference rather than seeing difference as grounds for discrimination or exploitation. Third, it is communalistic, not individualistic, especially valuing family and community over the individual in moral importance. Fourth, it is spiritual, not secular, rejecting any ultimate dichotomy of the sacred and the secular, acknowledging the pervasive presence and power of the unseen realm over and against what is seen. Fifth, it is theistic, not agnostic or atheistic, affirming not only the existence of God but also the relevance of belief to every aspect of life. Sixth, its basic approach or method is improvisational, not forced into fixed forms; it has an openness to spontaneity, flexibility and innovation, particularly in the realm of music and art. Seventh it is humanistic, not materialistic, valuing human life and dignity over material wealth or possessions.

These features of the African-American ethos are largely derived from traditional African cultures, yet it is important to bear in mind that in America as well as in Africa, this life-affirming perspective is not always strictly adhered to or applied. Nevertheless, the African-American ethos, notwithstanding many exceptions and abuses that can readily be cited, is essentially holistic, inclusive, communalistic, spiritual, theistic, improvisational, and humanistic in ways that the

Euro-American ethos is not, although exception would apply there also. Moreover, even if it is an exaggeration to say that the Euro-American ethos is dualistic, exclusive, individualistic, secular, atheistic, inflexible and materialistic, it must be recognized that these characteristics are necessary and sufficient conditions for the propagation of racism, which can be regarded as the logical consequence of a world view that readily expends both soul and spirit in pursuit of wealth.

Although the roots of the African-American ethos predate by centuries the exploitative schemes Europe brought to Africa, Asia, and the New World in the form of slavery, imperialism and colonialism, its best fruits are yet to emerge if and when African-Americans can resist the cultural and ethical assimilation of Euro-American values that have spelled death for our ancestors and our children; that is, if and when we can persuade ourselves and others to embrace African-American values that are humane and life-affirming.

THE PROBLEM OF A BLACK THEOLOGY

Black theology a term popularized some twenty years ago by Dr. James Cone, an African-American theologian and the author of *Black Theology and Black Power* (1969), is one of several specific cultural expressions of a broader genre known as "liberation theology." Liberation theologies all begin with the analysis of oppression, affirm the personhood of oppressed people, and advocate social and political change to liberate the oppressed. Black theology, in particular, analyzes the oppression of black people, affirms the personhood of black people, and advocates the social and political liberation of black people.

It is apparent that a strictly black or African-American theological perspective is limited. If there is only one God, in whose image all human beings are made, then reflections on the nature of God are severely restricted in any theological discourse that only takes account of the experience of one race, culture or gender. Yet the African-American experience provides an appropriate starting point, because all theological reflection is grounded in the particularities of race, class, gender, and culture. Indeed, all theologies have a contextual point of departure and may be rooted in the particularities of human experience, even if their ultimate conclusions point toward universal revelation and eschatological considerations. Therefore, the basic message and implications of black theology are not exclusive to the African-American community, though historically the experience of suffering, rejection, and exploitation in relation to the dominant culture has been a major hermeneutical concern of African-American religion. In other words, African-American religion never intended to isolate itself morally from the dominant culture but to stand as a witness against racism in the name of God. To the extent that blacks and whites identify themselves as Christians, the relevant scriptural mandate to love one's neighbor as oneself has been habitually violated— whites have despised their black neighbors, and blacks, insofar as they have internalized this racial hatred and animosity, have not loved themselves.

It is an established historical fact that the black churches emerged in response to racism not because African-Americans chose to exclude Euro-Americans from their worshiping communities, but because they were denied full participation in virtually every aspect of American life, including religion. Ironically the black churches were forced into existence by white churches that excluded blacks from participation in worship on the basis of racism and related ideas concerning the inferiority of African-American religion and culture on the one hand, and the superiority of Euro-American religion and culture on the other. It is tragic that racism overruled love in the justification of racial separation in the religious realm. And since the claim that Martin Luther King, Jr., made so many years ago, that 11:00 A.M. on Sunday morning is the most segregated hour in America, is still true, both black and white Christians must be held accountable for allowing racism, or the response to racism, to dictate their respective patterns of behavior and values systems in relation to each other.

While it may be valid to uphold the particular cultural traditions associated with religious worship, any theology that exclusively addresses the perspectives of one group without giving attention to the interests and concerns of others is suspect. It became characteristic of Euro-American religion to dichotomize and relativize any theological considerations that would question white hegemony. Rather than face the fact that slavery, terrorism, discrimination, and other manifestations of racism contradict the central teaching of the Christian faith—to love God and neighbor as oneself—it became more convenient and more consistent logically to invalidate any association between what one believes about God and what one does to others. While it is rare, even so, to find overt pronouncements of racist ideology in white religion, it seems understood by many that songs, sermons and liturgies about love of neighbor are not to be taken seriously with reference to black Christians. Praxis and principle are necessarily divorced from each other. On the other hand, it has historically been in the best interest of the African-American to lay full claim to the relevance of praxis to principle in a theological context in which God exercises sovereignty over all peoples in all situations— and not only during worship or on Sundays. It makes more sense to identify the separation of the sacred from the secular as an expression of the peculiarity or deviance of white religion than to single out the merger of the same as indicative of the distinctiveness of black religion. White Christianity and Judaism may be unique among the religions of the world in this regard.

In summary, if there is a distinctive perspective that black theology and black churches have brought to American life, it grows out of their courage to address questions of theodicy brought to the fore by the experience of racism, and their willingness to respond theologically to the reality of unmerited suffering. Black theology and the black churches consistently affirm the goodness of God, the evil capacities of humanity, and the promise of salvation offered through Jesus Christ to bring redemption, reconciliation, and wholeness to a broken world. Yet, the fact remains that any theology or any church whose existence is justified primarily on the basis of racism or its effects will bring serious deficiencies and liabilities to the dialogue needed to formulate a biomedical ethics that promotes justice, healing, and human dignity for all.

THE PROBLEM OF A BLACK ETHIC

The idea of a uniquely black ethic entails the same problems and limitations of black theology; it must transcend its particularity at some points in order to bring critical commentary to bear on the society at large. Although a number of ethicists and philosophers have sought to characterize the African-American ethic in comparison to and in contrast with its Euro-American counterpart, one of the most insightful analyses of the African-American ethic was published in 1971 Preston Williams, an African-American ethicist, in an article entitled "Ethics and Ethos in the Black Experience."[4] In it Williams offers a three-part typology to describe the life experiences of blacks in a racist America: (1) victimization, based on "the fact that every Black person in America is injured or cheated by the conscious and unconscious notions of white superiority in the American mind and social system"; (2) integration, achieved as an exception to the rule of racial exclusion by "the unusual Black who by the power of his intellect, drive or personality has forced his way into mainstream America in spite of the color of his skin"; and (3) black awareness, which goes "beyond integration to ask that all men recognize the existence of a spirit, a set of social structures and norms in Black life that are worthy of acquisition by Blacks and Whites."[5] Although all three aspects of this typology—victimization, integration, and black awareness—should be taken into account when evaluating the relevance of African-American ethical discourse to biomedical concerns, the fundamental assumption of the black awareness ideal, namely, that there are black values and norms that ought to be shared with and acquired by others, especially commends itself as a worthwhile point of departure for African-American participation in biomedical ethics.

Ultimately, the ethical question is not that of an African-American perspective but of African-American participation and inclusion. Perspective suggests a particular point of view, a unique angle or approach; participation assumes an unqualified stake and role within the whole discourse. It must not be forgotten that the hyphen in the term "African-American" connects two irreducible dimensions of experience: first, the retention of African identity, and second, the struggle for acceptance as Americans. Moreover, what is arguably the most distinctive ethical claim that African-Americans have made against a racist America, namely, the fundamental affirmation of human dignity regardless of social condition, is clearly worthy of acquisition by biomedical ethicists who are conscientiously concerned with transcending the particularities of race and culture in the pursuit of justice and human wholeness.

CAN BIOMEDICAL ETHICS BE ETHICAL?

An African-American perspective is ultimately a human perspective: a concrete, particular witness to universal truth. My conclusion is that in order to be truly ethical, biomedical ethics must be holistic, inclusive, communalistic and humanistic, if not also spiritual, theistic and improvisational; that is, it ought to reflect both the particularity and universality of the African-American ethos. This ethos should not be regarded as merely an interesting minority perspective or contribution, but should inform the shape and content of the whole discourse. It follows that this ethos can serve as a rich resource for research and dialogue with regard to pressing issues such as health-care resource allocation, treatment or non-treatment decisions, patient and physician relationships, and the management of reproductive technologies and interventions. Finally, it is my conviction that any biomedical ethics that does not give priority to justice and human dignity in the administration of health care is unethical, regardless of the racial identity or cultural context of the persons involved.

NOTES

1. Harley Flack and Edmund D. Pellegrino, "New Data Suggests African-Americans Have Own Perspective on Biomedical Ethics," Kennedy Institute of Ethics *Newsletter* 3:2 (April 1989): 2.

2. I prefer to use the term "Euro-American" in place of "Anglo-American" because it compares more consistently with "African-American" in reference to contingents of origin, and it avoids the typically American bias that regards "Anglo" as superior to or representative of the rest of Europe.

3. Flack and Pellegrino, "New Data Suggests," 1.

4. Preston N. Williams, "Ethics and Ethos n the Black Experience," *Christianity and Crisis*, 31 May 1971: 104-105.

5. Ibid.

JAMES E. BOWMAN

The Plight of Poor African-Americans: Public Policy on Sickle Hemoglobins and AIDS

Unprecedented advances in health biotechnology have not been translated to improvement in health care for poor African-Americans. It is well to be constantly reminded of this assertion while the West celebrates the "End of History." Fukuyama coined that phrase this year to claim the triumph of the West, of the Western idea, over that of communist ideology. He stated:

> What we may be witnessing is not just the end of the Cold War, or the passing of a particular period of postwar history, but the end of history as such: that is, the end point of man's ideological evolution and the universalization of Western liberal democracy as the final form of human government.[1]

But is the final form of human government to sanction homelessness for thousands of individuals and families—the freedom to live under bridges and beg in the streets—and poverty for one-third or more of African-Americans? Is it to have inadequate to nonexistent health care for millions of Americans and a maternal and infant mortality rate among African-Americans that is the highest infant mortality rate in the major industrialized countries and worse than Cuba's? Consequently, the declaration of "the end to history" is yet another reminder to African-Americans that they are the forgotten, the hidden blight.

In a reply to Fukuyama, Himmelfarb elaborated on Fukuyama's claim that the future of liberal democracy is assured because it has succeeded in resolving the "class issue" and that the social problems that remain, such as black poverty, are not a function of liberalism but the historical legacy of premodern conditions: slavery and racism. Himmelfarb argues that even if this were so, the problems remain and continue to plague us, while solutions evade us. "History," he writes, "has a habit of bequeathing to us disastrous legacies, bombs that can explode at any time and any place."[2] Himmelfarb believed that black poverty and the poverty of the underclass is not the relic of an old problem but a new problem, and that black poverty may be subversive because liberal democracy does not understand it, let alone cope with it. Himmelfarb's thesis is ominous, for if the quandary of black poverty does not fit into the ideology of liberal democracy, and if there is no solution for it, violence and repression will follow.

Ideology and mythology pervade political decision making about health care priorities. Habermas and members of the Frankfurt School of critical theory expose "ideological delusion" and avow that modern industrial societies exercise such extensive control over even the inner life of their members that they prevent them from becoming fully aware that they are frustrated and miserable.[3] Witness a common shibboleth: health care resources are scarce. This pronouncement is a national disgrace and an ethical perversion: economists, politicians, scientists, philosophers, and physicians claim without a flicker of remorse that decent health care for all is impossible in our democracy. I, for one, would not want to go to sleep under the care of a physician who espoused such a position.

Health care is facilitated and complicated by spectacular advances in biotechnology. Nevertheless, while we embrace new technology, African-Americans must be aware that historians, philosophers, scientists, physicians, politicians, jurists, and educators have often used scientific advances as weapons for their own nefarious ends under the privileged mantle of scholarship. We can examine some facets of sickle hemoglobin as a model for caution in this regard.

SICKLE CELL DISEASE AND SICKLE CELL TRAIT

Sickle cell disease is an inherited disorder of hemoglobin (the oxygen-carrying protein of blood) in which, under conditions of reduced oxygen tension, the red cells assume the form of a sickle. This results in the plugging of blood vessels with subsequent damage to tissue or organs. The most common sites affected are the lungs, liver, kidneys, brain, heart, and hips. The life expectancy is quite variable and unpredictable, unlike that of Tay-Sachs disease. Some individuals with sickle cell disease die at an early age; some are intermittently ill throughout a short or long life; others reach adulthood without knowing that they have the disorder; a few live late into the seventh decade of life.

The carrier state is termed "sickle cell trait" (hemoglobin AS). Medical reports often associate sickle cell trait with sudden death. A study of Armed Forces recruits showed an increased incidence of death during or following vigorous exercise associated with dehydration.[4] Yet some of our best football and track athletes have sickle cell trait and perform in the high altitudes of Denver (5,000 feet) and Mexico City (7,500) without difficulty.[5]

Occasionally a person with sickle cell trait may have rare episodes of blood in the urine, but an overwhelming majority do not. In the early days of sickle hemoglobin testing, many physicians, community groups, and publications from the National Institutes of Health did not delineate sickle cell trait from sickle cell disease. The confusion of sickle cell trait with sickle cell disease was undoubtedly the principal basis for the flood of early mandatory state sickle cell hemoglobin legislation.[6]

DISTRIBUTION OF SICKLE HEMOGLOBIN IN POPULATIONS

Sickle hemoglobin is found in high frequency in peoples of African origin, in Southern Italians (particularly Sicilians), Greeks, Eti-Turks, Arabs, Egyptians, Eastern Jews, Southern Iranians, and Asiatic Indians.[7] In the United States about 8 percent of African-Americans have sickle cell trait; about one in 500 black newborns have sickle cell disease, and approximately 45,000 African-Americans have sickle cell disease.

SICKLE CELL ANEMIA PROGRAMS

Sickle cell anemia education, testing, and counseling programs in the United States have developed in three phases: (1) mass population education, testing, and counseling of children, adolescents, adults, and couples before and after marriage; (2) newborn screening; and (3) prenatal diagnosis. These three stages followed the development of new technology, and predictably, new technology necessitated alterations in policy.

Several articles and monographs have outlined the course of events leading to the sickle cell anemia programs of the early 1970s.[8]

Sickle cell programs were prompted by the making of a commercial test for the presence of sickle hemoglobin produced by Ortho-Pharmaceutical Corporation and later altered by many other companies. This test was advertised as a test for sickle hemoglobin, but it did not differentiate sickle cell trait from sickle cell disease. Community and other lay groups and even physicians began mass genetic screening programs using only the solubility tests. Some groups counseled that sickle cell trait was a mild form of sickle cell disease. Unknowledgeable physicians asserted that patients who had sickle cell anemia would not live past early childhood or would be dead by the age of twenty. Spurious and reputable sickle cell anemia organizations were created nationwide. Thousands of dollars were raised for mass screening with inappropriate tests; individuals were often improperly counseled by physicians and lay persons who were swayed by the propaganda. Consequently, legislators were pressed to pass mandatory sickle hemoglobin screening laws by persons who erroneously believed that one in twelve black Americans had a disease the would kill them before age twenty. Unfortunately, the stigma and misinformation about sickle cell trait and sickle cell disease is almost as prevalent today as it was in the early 1970s.

A shocking example (from late 1987) will illustrate this assertion. A man was beaten unconscious with a large flashlight by police and left unattended for about five hours in jail. The prisoner was finally taken to the hospital and died soon thereafter. At postmortem, sickling was found in the blood vessels; subsequently it was determined that the man had sickle cell crisis, but the medical examiner did not know that intravascular sickling is often found in surgical and postmortem specimens from persons with sickle cell trait—after all, there is no greater anoxia than death.[9] In a study of coroner's cases in Cook County, Illinois, Kirschner and Bowman found intravascular sickling in all postmortems of individuals with sickle cell trait who died from trauma.[10] I have been consulted on many such cases, beginning in the 1970s. Since the advent of the article associating sickle cell trait with sudden death, I have had a flood of consultations about persons with sickle cell trait who die after having been beaten or given sedatives. Do persons with sickle cell trait die after being bludgeoned or anesthetized? Of course they do. Persons who do not have sickle cell trait also die following trauma or sedation. Individuals with sickle cell trait may be relatively resistant to falciparum malaria, but not death. The erroneous association of postmortem intravascular sickling with sickle cell trait has technically led to legalized murder of persons with sickle cell trait.[11] Physicians now attempt to avoid justifiable malpractice claims of wrongful death, by quoting an Armed Forces study in support of their misdiagnoses.[12]

The contention is that the main design of sickle cell education, testing, and counseling programs is informed decision making about sickle hemoglobin. This shibboleth conceals the obvious: it is inconceivable that Congress would have allocated approximately 80 million health dollars since 1972 for nationwide screening and education clinics, subsidy for state newborn screening for sickle cell disease, and demonstration education, testing and counseling components of Comprehensive Sickle Cell Centers, if they did not believe—or had not been led to believe—that federal funding for education, testing, and counseling would lead to a significant decrease in the number of children with sickle cell disease and a consequent saving in health care costs. In fact, the Federal Legislation that authorized the National Sickle Cell Disease Program was called the "National Sickle Cell Anemia Control Act." Nevertheless, the educational, social, and economic blight in the poor black community obviates almost any large scale community genetics program and will also compromise a community AIDS program, no matter how well conceived. A central impediment to these programs is out-of-wedlock births.[13]

Societal forces in the black community within the past twenty years have resulted in an increase in out-of-wedlock births from 20 percent to 80 percent in some urban areas. Yet, sickle cell and other genetics education, testing, and counseling programs often emphasize the importance of testing before marriage. Unfortunately, this premise ignores an important reality: children are born as a result of mating, not marriage.

OUT OF WEDLOCK BIRTHS

Wilson's group at the University of Chicago analyzed problems of out-of-wedlock births in the black community as part of a large scale investigation of the tragedy of the "black underclass."[14] Wilson contended that the striking increase in the proportion of out-of-wedlock births was a major factor in the rise of families in the black community headed by females. The growth in the number of births outside of marriage is indicative of trends in fertility and marital status and also of changes in population composition. Not only has the incidence of premarital conception increased, but the proportion of premarital pregnancies that were legitimated by marriage has decreased. Accordingly, out-of-wedlock births today constitute a much greater proportion of total births than they did in the past. Interestingly, Wilson asserts that the black out-of-wedlock birth ratio has increased precipitously, not because the rate of extramarital births has significantly increased, but because the percentage of women married and the rate of marital fertility have both declined. Further, the decrease in the proportion of women who are married and living with their husbands reflects both a sharp rise in separation and divorce rates and a considerable increase in the percentage of "never-married women." These figures have been particularly striking for black women; the proportion of black women married and living with their husbands decreased from 52 percent in 1947 to 34 percent in 1980. To compound the problem, Wilson showed that the proportion of never-married Black women increased from 65 percent in 1965 to 82 percent in 1980 for those ages fourteen to twenty-four, and from 8 percent to 21 percent for ages twenty-five to forty-four.

Wilson then analyzed changes in the age structure that have contributed to the differential in out-of-wedlock births in the black community. In 1960, 36 percent of black women ages fifteen to forty-four were between fifteen to twenty-four years of age. However, by 1975 the proportion had increased to 46 percent, and the comparable increase for white women was from 34 to 42 percent in 1975. Accordingly, Wilson concluded that changes in the age structure increase the proportion of births occurring to young women, result in higher out-of-wedlock birth ratios among young black women, and inflate the proportion of all births that occur outside of marriage.

The increase in families headed by females has disastrous social and economic consequences because such families are much more vulnerable to poverty than are others.[15] Wilson pointed out that the poverty rate of families headed by females was 36.3 percent in 1982, but the rate for married-couple families was only 7.6 percent Finally, Wilson indicated that the increasingly critical jobless rate for black males also contributes to the out-of-wedlock birth rate, for an obvious reason: black women see little advantage in marrying a man who is unlikely to contribute to family support.

Any genetics program in the black community that does not take these social and economic factors into consideration will have almost no prospect for success. It is inconceivable that under such conditions there will be reproductive restraint not to produce children with sickle cell disease. At the same time, tragic economic and social conditions in the black community could serve as a focus for the resurgence of eugenics programs among the poor and black with the almost irrefutable rationale of saving health care costs.

Accordingly, any health program, genetic or otherwise, that does not include a commitment to ameliorate poverty, improve education of the poor, or create jobs in the black community will be a mockery. Then, as usual, the victims will be blamed, and more draconian measures will follow.

A FEDERAL PROPOSAL TO MANDATE
NEWBORN SCREENING

In April 1987, "A National Institutes of Health Consensus Development Conference Statement on Newborn Screening for Sickle Cell Disease and Other Hemoglobinopathies" recommended universal screening of all newborns for hemoglobinopathies. This is the first time that a federal panel recommended mandated testing for a genetic disorder. The panel asserted that the health risks to children with sickle cell disease are so great that major efforts must be made to identify every affected child; but for those states with very few at-risk members, targeted screening should be considered.

The panel also advised that prenatal and neonatal screening as a continuum of care be instituted. This recommendation would make prenatal diagnosis possible but, as expected, the panel was *loudly silent* on the next step: abortion of affected fetuses. The word abortion is taboo in federal, most state, and even national, privately funded genetics programs, because directors of these programs fear that "right to life" groups will target them for extinction.

Not only did the panel stress universal screening; it was also unequivocal on voluntary versus mandated screening. The panel emphasized: "The benefits of screening are so compelling that its provision should not be left to the discretion of individual physicians or health care facilities."[16]

Newborn screening for sickle cell disease, however, must not be dissociated from a holistic health policy. If we ask poor mothers to participate in newborn and prenatal screening programs for genetic disorders or any other disease, but do not fight for universal prenatal care, equitable health care delivery, education, adequate housing, and food, then we are co-conspirators in health care deception.

PRENATAL DIAGNOSIS

The county hospitals of the State of California were ordered in 1988 not to admit pregnant women to their clinics for prenatal care unless the pregnant women had appropriate health insurance or sufficient funds.[17] Yet, the State of California has one of the most comprehensive prenatal screening programs for neural tube defects in the

United States.[18] Other prenatal genetic screening for a variety of genetic disorders is widely available. The denial of prenatal care in county hospitals in California is a perversion of health care: maternal and infant mortality will consequently increase. Newborn screening and prenatal diagnosis for a variety of genetic disorders is discouraged.

The prenatal diagnosis of sickle cell disease is compromised by many factors, the most important of which is prenatal care. How can a mother whose child or children have died because of a callous health care system be enthusiastic about a program of prenatal diagnosis? Predictably, recent health statistics show that large differentials exist by race, with black mothers receiving early prenatal care less frequently than white mothers in all states.[19] Over 70 percent of white mothers received early prenatal care in all but two states. However, less than 70 percent of black mothers received early prenatal care in twenty of the twenty-seven states (including the District of Columbia) with black populations of 150,000 or more. The rate is especially low (less than 55 percent) for black women in four southern states, Florida, Kentucky, Arkansas, Oklahoma, and in New York.

Access to prenatal care is not the only barrier to prenatal diagnosis for genetic disorders. Although *Roe v. Wade*[20] sanctioned abortion under certain conditions, *Maher v. Roe*[21] and *Harris v. McRae* ruled that even though women had a right to an abortion, the State is under no obligation to pay for it.[22] Nevertheless, federal funds are used to support research in genetics programs and techniques for prenatal diagnosis. *Scientists are supported but poor women are not.* Consequently, programs for prenatal diagnosis for sickle cell disease, and other disorders, including AIDS, will be compromised by a public policy that takes poor women to the brink and then offers them no assistance—except in the few states that authorize public funding for abortion.

But is abortion such an anathema in the black community that programs that lead to abortion will be unsuccessful? Unfortunately, there have been no prospective studies in sickle cell programs that were designed with the intent of answering this important question. In an investigation of disease, Driscoll et. al. found that of eleven fetuses predicted to have sickle cell anemia, six were terminated.[23] Nevertheless, studies of referred cases are from a biased sample. But AIDS has far more serious consequences than does sickle cell disease, and the acceptance of abortion for affected fetuses is predictably related to the severity of the disease.

A clue to the acceptability of abortion in the black community may be gained from a review of abortion statistics.[24] Legal abortions are now a significant method of birth control. In the white population, the number of abortions per hundred live births was 17.5 percent in 1973 and 31.2 percent in 1981. Blacks constituted the vast majority of the "all others" group. In this group the abortions per hundred live births in 1973 was 28.9 and in 1981, 54.4. These figures are instructive because contrary to common belief, a significant proportion of an underprivileged group manages to obtain abortions. On the other hand these figures could indicate that middle and upper-income black women disproportionately elect abortion as an aid to birth control, but this premise is unlikely.

CONSEQUENCES OF EARLY STATE AND COMMUNITY SICKLE HEMOGLOBIN PROGRAMS

There are lessons to be learned from misguided sickle hemoglobin programs that were instituted in the early 1970s. These programs led to: (1) stigmatization of potentially two million African-Americans with sickle cell trait; (2) mandatory sickle hemoglobin screening laws in twelve states (including the District of Columbia); some were quite subtle, others were not. Massachusetts passed the first law, with Arizona, Georgia, Illinois, Kentucky, Louisiana, Maryland, Mississippi, New Mexico, New York, and Virginia to follow; (3) increased insurance rates for persons with sickle cell trait, even though morbidity and mortality in this group is not significantly different from those who do not have sickle cell trait; (4) the firing of flight attendants with sickle cell trait; (5) rejection of persons with sickle cell trait from flight and other hazardous service in the Armed Forces; (6) the banning of persons with sickle cell trait from athletics, even though some of the best football, basketball, and track athletes have sickle cell trait and compete effectively at high altitudes; and (7) sterilization of carriers of sickle hemoglobin.[25]

Once it becomes general knowledge that the birth of children with certain genetic disorders is preventable, other members of the family and the community may question why women at risk for having children with severe disorders persist in having children. If poor women persist in bearing children with preventable severe disorders, regulation of reproduction by the state does not have to be so indecent as to require mandatory sterilization (which is constitutional), abortion, or prenatal diagnosis. A more subtle, indirect and coercive edict is available. The Supreme Court in *Dandridge v. Williams* upheld the legality of a welfare grant by the State of Maryland regulation that restricted total Aid for Dependent Children (AFDC) to a maximum of $250 per month, no matter how large the family.[26] If restrictions on welfare payments for healthy children have been upheld by the highest Court of the land, an extension of this precedent to include the interdiction of the birth of poor children with severe genetic disorders by edict or by covert duress logically follows. Poor children with genetic disorder or AIDS are far more costly to the state than are poor, deprived, malnourished children without genetic diseases or AIDS.

AIDS

The tragedy of the underclass in the black community has been exacerbated by AIDS. Although some of the errors of sickle cell programs may be applicable to public health efforts to prevent AIDS, there are important differences. AIDS is a communicable disease that is virtually 100 percent fatal. Sickle cell disease is a genetic disorder with a variable life expectancy. Unfortunately, federal, state, and voluntary efforts to "control" sickle cell disease have employed the principle of the "police power" of the state to effect mandatory genetics programs such as those used for communicable diseases. Such programs are one of the many causes of stigmatization of persons with sickle cell trait and sickle cell disease. The health care costs for a child with sickle cell disease could exceed those of persons with AIDS, because individuals with sickle cell disease live longer.

AIDS is a deadly, communicable disease, and the health care costs may exceed $100,000 per year per patient, but once the disease is manifest, life expectancy is short. On the other hand, the number of AIDS patients produces a severe strain on the health care system. Weinberg and Murray report that in New York City in 1987, over 1000 beds, about 5 percent of the total acute-care beds, were occupied continually by about four thousand patients with AIDS.[27] These authors estimated that by 1991 about 25 to 50 percent of New York City's medical-surgical beds will be constantly occupied by patients with AIDS. Additional pertinent figures from Weinberg and Murray suggest that four to five hundred thousand New Yorkers may carry HIV; the prevalence of HIV antibodies within an estimated population of five hundred thousand male homosexuals is about 50 percent; and seropositive individuals within the two hundred thousand drug abuse population may be anywhere from 50 to 87 percent.

Interestingly, the male homosexual community has been effective in preventing the labeling of AIDS as a communicable disease in California, in order to prevent the tracing of contacts. The penalty for unauthorized disclosure of the results of testing includes a fine of ten thousand dollars and a jail sentence of up to two years. Accordingly, California physicians do not share the information with their colleagues or record the results on the chart, even if they are negative.[28] Consequently, AIDS is medically communicable, but politically noncommunicable. This anachronism is public policy because the white male homosexual community is well organized, generally well educated, politically astute, and exercises its right to vote. Haber thus alleges that AIDS is the first politically protected pandemic in the history of the world.[29]

What about pregnant women who are at high risk for AIDS? If draconian laws and measures have already been instituted for a genetic disorder with a variable life expectancy such as sickle cell disease, programs to prevent AIDS in newborns will be more coercive. Shaw castigates women who knowingly have severely affected children that could have been prevented by prenatal diagnosis and abortion.[30] Shaw's will probably be one of many similar proposals in the future. Compulsory AIDS prevention programs will be easier to institute because AIDS in newborns in major urban ghettos is primarily found in pregnant women who are themselves intravenous drug addicts or whose partners are similar addicts. Poor African-American or Hispanic women who are addicts have triple indemnity and are thus highly vulnerable. Those who live on the edge of society have few defenders. For example, Haber asserts that

> The intravenous drug users apparently have an unmanageable suicidal drive. If they won't modify their behavior, knowing the way in which drugs destroy their minds or knowing of the strong possibility of dying immediately of a drug overdose, then the possibility of AIDS in about a half a dozen years isn't going to have any great effect. Unfortunately, they share their infections with their heterosexual partners. Homosexuals and bisexuals know their risks, and although subpopulations of them are already infected, many of them continue their unsafe practices.[31]

No matter what experts in their wisdom decide, AIDS will continue to be a major problem in the underclass unless we begin to ameliorate the blatant inequalities that are the basic cause of impoverishment in the midst of affluence. On the other hand, poor African-American and Hispanic women who are drug addicts—or whose partners are addicts—produce large numbers of children with a fatal, preventable disease that is rightfully feared by the majority of Americans. The intravenous drug subculture has no political clout.

I want now to examine the problem of the prevention of AIDS in newborns. Should all pregnant women be tested, or should only women in high risk communities be tested, or should only African-American and Hispanic women in high risk communities be examined? And should the testing be mandatory or voluntary?

Some vital population and AIDS statistics may be helpful. In 1981 the total live births in the United States were 3,629,238 of which 2,908,669 were white; 587,797 were black; and the remainder unclassified.[32] The best general population statistics have been obtained from military recruits, although an extremely biased sample. The army screened for HIV infection in more than 640,000 civilians who applied for military service. In this sample, black men between the ages of twenty-one and twenty-five had an estimated infection rate of 1 in 210 to 1 in 350 per year. White males in the same sample had an HIV prevalence rate of 1 in 1,000 to 1 in 5,000 per year.

A prenatal testing program to decrease the incidence of the birth of children with AIDS would include counseling, follow-up, out-patient and hospital patient care. Out-patient and hospital costs were, unfortunately, never included in sickle cell federal programs nor in any of the state-mandated programs. Children and newborns, as well as adults with sickle cell diseases were found, but cost of care has always been left to our deficient health care system.

If we were to screen all pregnant women for AIDS, and if the price of testing, confirmatory testing, and counseling are very conservatively estimated at $100 per woman, the cost per year would be in excess of 370 million dollars. Added to this figure would be the cost for abortions for women who screened positive and health care costs for those who appeared for prenatal care too late for abortion or who refused abortion. To this should be added the voluntary follow-up of the sexual partners, though this could entail the tracing of sexual contacts for at least the previous ten years. I also have not factored into this estimate the costs of education, training, and the certification of counselors. Needless to say, this approach does not appear feasible in terms of cost—or personnel availability. But it may be. A distinguished group of scientists and physicians in Great Britain have suggested that all pregnant women in that country be screened for AIDS.[33]

Should only African-American and Hispanic women from high risk regions be tested? This would be the cheapest but also the most discriminatory of plans. It is unlikely in light of the deplorable health care available to poor African-Americans and Hispanics that leaders in those communities would countenance restrictive testing of this nature. Effective education, testing, and counseling programs must have community support. On the other hand, the sickle hemoglobin model is instructive. African-American leaders initiated and encouraged mandatory testing of African-Americans for sickle hemoglobin with disastrous results. They were guided by misinformation.[34] Even so, it would be callous public policy to instigate mandatory testing programs without first attempting to ameliorate some of the social causes of AIDS in high risk, heterosexual groups.

Meanwhile, children are born with AIDS in places that can least afford this added burden, and with the prospect of 100 percent mortality. This is needless suffering in a community where even salvageable children are dying because of a social, economic, educational, and political system that ignores the poor. American human rights activists travel far and wide ferreting out human rights violations abroad, and ignoring the ultimate human rights violations at home: social and political neglect of the plight of poor children in the United States.

If HIV testing of pregnant women is to be done, and if the tests are accurate enough so that a false positive rate is virtually nonexistent—and there is some doubt on the point[35]—another approach to consider would be voluntary testing of all pregnant women in high risk regions of the United States. We already screen newborn African-American children for phenylketonuria and for cystic fibrosis but these disorders are quite rare in African-Americans. We do newborn screening for some genetic disorders in which the prevalence is as low as one in one hundred thousand newborns. Therefore why not screen even so-called "low-risk groups" in high risk communities. In fact, the equal protection clause of the Fourteenth Amendment of the Constitution might insure that screening not be selective or discriminatory. But the doctrine which holds that the public interest of the state supersedes the private interest of individuals was reiterated in the landmark Supreme Court decision of *Munn v. Illinois*.[36] Although these utilitarian precepts are common to most societies, they have also led to some of our most restrictive state legislation.

I suspect that we will legislate mandatory AIDS testing for high risk pregnant women. A one in fifty incidence of AIDS antibodies in an African-American and Hispanic community like that of New York cannot be ignored.[37] Nevertheless, I doubt that we will legislate mandatory equitable education, decent housing, health care for all, or full employment. The ghettos will remain, and the only people who will benefit will be the army of administrators, public health experts, and health care and social workers who will plan, oversee, and execute the program. But AIDS in poor children will persist, because we will address the symptoms but not the fundamental causes of inequitable distribution of health care in this the most affluent of countries.

NOTES

1.   F. Fukuyama, "The End of History? *The National Interest* 16:4.

2.   G. Himmelfarb, "Response to the End of History?" *The National Interest*, 16:24-26.

3.   R. Gress, *The Idea of a Critical Theory: Habermas and the Frankfurt School* (Cambridge: Cambridge University Press, 1988).

4.   Ibid.

5.   J. E. Bowman, "Ethical, Legal, and Humanistic Implications of Sickle Cell Programs," INSERM 44:278-353.

6.   Ibid.; See also J. E. Bowman, "Genetic Screening Programs and Public Policy" *Phylon* 38:117-142.

7.   J. E. Bowman, "Ethical, Legal, and Humanistic Implications," 278-353.

8.   Ibid.; See also J. E. Bowman, "Genetic Screening Program," *Phylon* 38:117-142; J. E. Bowman, "Mass Screening Programs for Sickle Hemoglobin: A Sickle Cell Crisis," *The Journal of the American Medical Association* 222:1650 and P. Reilly, *Genetics, Law, and Social Policy* (Cambridge: Harvard University Press, 1977).

9.   J. E. Bowman, "Ethical, Legal and Humanistic Implications," INSERM 44:278-353.

10. R. H. Kirschner and J. E. Bowman, "The Sickle Cell Trait Sudden Death Fallacy," *1980 Proceedings of the Annual Meeting of the American Academy of Forensic Science.*

11.   Bowman, "Ethical, Legal, and Humanistic Implications of Sickle Cell Programs," INSERM 44:278-353 and "Genetic Screening Programs and Public Policy," PHYLON 38:117-142.

12.   J. A. Kark et.al., "Sickle Cell Trait As a Risk Factor for Sudden Death in Physical Training" *The New England Journal of Medicine* 317:781-787.

13.   J. E. Bowman, "Is a National Program to Prevent Sickle Cell Disease Possible?" *The American Journal of Pediatric Hematology/Oncology* 5 (Winter 1983): 362-372.

14.   W. J. Wilson, *The Truly Disadvantaged: The Inner City, The Underclan, and Public Policy* (Chicago: The University of Chicago Press, 1987).

15.   Ibid.

16.   "A Natural Institutes of Health Consensus Development Conference Statement on Newborn Screening for Sickle Cell Disease and Other Hemoglobinopathies," The National Institute of Health, April, 1987.

17.   This was communicated personally to me by G. C. Cunningham.

18.   R. Steinbrook, "In California: Voluntary Mass Prenatal Screening," *The Hastings Center Report* 16:5-7.

19.   "Health in the United States," Department of Health and Human Services Publication No. (PHS) 85-1232, (1987).

20.   Roe v. Wade 410 U.S. 116, 1973.

21.   Maher v. Roe 432 U.S. 464, 1973.

21.   Harris v. McRae 48 *Law Week*, 4941, 1980.

22. M.C. Driscoll et.al., "Prenatal Diagnosis of Sickle Hemaglobinopathies: The Experience of the Columbia University Comprehensive Center for Sickle Cell Disease" in *The American Journal of Human Genetics* 40:548-558.

23. See note 13 above.

24. See note 11 above and J. E. Bowman, "Mass Screening Programs for Sickle Hemoglobin: A Sickle Cell Crisis," *The Journal of the American Medical Association* 222:1650.

25. See note 11 above and J. E. Bowman, "Mass Screening Programs for Sickle Hemoglobin: A Sickle Cell Crisis," *The Journal of the American Medical Association* 222:1650.

26. Dandridge v. Williams 397 U.S. 471, 485, 1970.

27. D. S. Weinberg and H. W. Murray, "Coping With AIDS," *The New England Journal of Medicine* 317:1469-1472.

28. S. L. Haber in "The Four Fatal Myths of AIDS" in *CAP TODAY* (August 1987): 5-6.

29. Ibid.

30. M. W. Shaw, "Conditional Prospective Rights of the Fetus" *The Journal of Legal Medicine* 5:63-115.

31. See note 28 above.

32. See note 19 above.

33. D. W. Black et.al., "HIV Testing of All Pregnant Women," *Lancet* ii:1277.

34. See note 25 above.

35. D. B. Barnes, "New Questions About AIDS Test Accuracy," *Science* 238: 884-885.

36. Munn v. Illinois 97 U.S. 124, 1876.

37. S. Landesman et.al., "Serosurvey of Human Immunodeficiency Virus Infection in Partrurients," *The Journal of the American Medical Association* 258:2701-2703.

William A. Banner

Is There an African-American Perspective on Biomedical Ethics? The View from Philosophy

Any attention to human difference or diversity and any talk about *ethnic perspective* in medical science and in ethics brings to the fore the historic *problem of universals*, that is, the question whether a common term, such as *man* or *human*, designates a distinct *kind* of thing or merely applies conveniently to apparent similarities among discrete individual entities. Aristotle, who was the son of a physician and initially a marine biologist (after leaving Plato's Academy), distinguished, in one of his logical treatises (*Topics*), the *terms* of discourse as employed in attribution, namely, *definition*, *property*, *genus*, and *accident*. Of these, *definition* indicates the essence of a thing (το τι ην ειναι), i.e., what a thing is as a *kind* of thing, especially a natural kind.[1] Human beings are recognizable as a *kind* by morphological similarities and by generation and descent. Man as a distinct kind of being is separate from all other kinds of things; and *man* begets man (ανθρωπος ανθρωπον γεννα).[2]

If with Aristotle one is to take *classification* seriously and accept the essential *uniformity* of human life, then one must recognize human diversity as variation occurring along with the manifestation of the same form or formal nature. In other words, diversity—however broad or extensive—is the manifestation of form or kind or type together with the *concrete individuality* of "numerable" things. One encounters immediately and directly the individual thing and one comes to grasp the *form* (as well as nonformal features) common to many individuals. The particularities of human life are either inherited or acquired. Particularity separates individual from individual and group from group without displacing or obscuring the *defining* characters of human life as a *kind* of existence.

In the modern anthropological debate, either human diversity is seen as compatible with human uniformity or what has been called

188

the "unity of mankind," or human diversity is seen as opposing and displacing uniformity, leaving discreetness as the only object of the empirical description of human life.

In the eighteenth century Georges Buffon opposed the idea of uniformity in nature, declaring that all classifications by genera and species embrace "something arbitrary."[3] There are simply no clear-cut differences in nature; genera and species are only figments or creatures of the imagination. Buffon regarded himself, along with Pierre Maupertis, as an evolutionist; and it is clear that in 1749 he held a view of nature and of natural history that anticipated in many respects the general position of Charles Darwin a century later. For it can be said that the real posture of Darwin's *Origin of Species*, published in 1859, is the *denial* of species or kinds: "there is no fallible criterion," Darwin maintained, "by which to distinguish species and well-marked varieties."[4] Darwin says further on this point: "I look at individual differences . . . as being the first step toward . . . varieties and at varieties as leading to sub-species, and to species."[5]

Darwin was apparently satisfied that the interaction between living things and their environment is such as to produce incalculable variations, the persistence of some of which would be a function of natural "selection." Darwin allows at the same time that it is possible that "individuals of the same species . . . have within a not remote period descended from one parent, and have migrated from some one birthplace."[6]

The emphasis on human variation and diversity was given currency in modern times by the efforts of scientists as well as nonscientists to embrace anthropological information arising in part from the contacts of Europeans with non-Europeans. The poet and philosopher, Johannn Gottfried Herder, writing in 1787 in *Ideas on the Philosophy of History*, saw human variation as the direct result of environmental influence, an influence yielding over a period of time distinct species or subspecies differing not only physically but also in temperament and in moral disposition.[7] Herder was eloquent in his affirmation of the oneness of mankind and the unity of all persons, yet he apparently found the "evidence" of human diversity convincing and even overwhelming. The eminent unity of Herder and others fostered, however inadvertently, the modern popular idea of "racial types" as discrete human categories. Joseph de Maistre, polemicist and opponent of the French Revolution, said in 1797: "I have seen, in my time, Frenchmen, Italians, Russians, . . . But as for Man, I declare I have never met him in my life; if he exists, it is without my knowledge."[8] De Maistre thus heralds the racial or ethnic particularism that has dominated the thought and action of the nineteenth and twentieth centuries.

The question now before us is whether the idea of ethnic particularism as carried over into medical ethics is tenable or untenable and fatuous. The question remains the same whether one employs the term "race" (meaning the persistence of certain physical traits, in generation and descent, as the basis for "consciousness of kind" and distinctness of culture) or the term "ethnic" (with its broader sociological meaning of "any number of people accustomed to living together" or "any number of people regarded in a society as constituting a group distinct from the dominant group and distinct from other groups").

One is brought to ask what precisely is the object of thought and action in dealing with problems from a racial or ethnic *perspective*. The medical concern for the physical and mental well-being of persons would seem to be a *universally* unlimited concern. And the ethical responsibility for good judgment and justice in human affairs would seem to be a *universally* unlimited responsibility. How indeed does one avoid the broadest "field of view" in such matters?

How, for example, does the cancer of the pancreas incurred by an African-American differ, as an object of medical concern, from the cancer of the pancreas incurred by a Greek-American or Anglo-American? Surely there is a definition and knowledge of cancer or of pancreatic cancer that covers the disease of both African-Americans and Greek-Americans, although the precise features of the disease and the precise circumstances of its incidence may vary from group to group and from person to person.

It should be clear that when the focus of attention is on a precisely definable problem, one encounters an extramental, extrapersonal order of things to which the term "perspective" is inapplicable or inappropriate. In their concern with the maintenance and restoration of health, physicians, other medical persons, and their advisors are involved in bringing the best medical resources within the reach of the community as a whole. If it were an epidemiological fact that only white persons have suffered from cystic fibrosis and only black persons have suffered from sickle-cell anemia, no *ethnic* perspective would be pertinent to the appreciation of the matter at hand. What is pertinent is the bearing of medical knowledge and research on our understanding of a manifest human disability and the genetic, physiology, social, and environmental circumstances attending its incidence. It is pertinent to see a medical disability as a human disability or predicament having discoverable causal conditions and having probably repeatable manifestations in other persons or groups under the same or similar conditions.

My position, in summary, is that the conduct of the science of medicine or the conduct of the science of ethics is incompatible with anything called "ethnic perspective." Analysis, both in medical science and in ethics, is an affair of critical intelligence. Such intelligence operates at both the general and the particular levels, i.e., it gives attention to the common in human existence and experience as well as to the individual or proper "in that experience." Aristotle devotes Book I of his *Parts of Animals* to methodology in the life sciences. And it is Aristotle who points out the *error of redundancy* in investigation, i.e., the error of considering a matter or matters at the lower (specific) level and ignoring the higher (generic) level of morphological and causal factors that govern diverse particular instances of the same phenomenon. The cost of this redundancy is the time and effort spent in treating as discrete and isolated matters that fall under the same common notion or notions, and thus repeating the same description and analysis over and over again.

The universality of science and ethics is the answer to racism and to the prejudice and insensitivity that have followed in the wake of racism. Whatever ethnic and social divisions there are in our society and in the world, one must say that there is only one medical community, which addresses itself to the alleviation of physical and mental discomfort and disease, and only one ethical or moral community, which addresses itself to the responsibilities of good judgment, justice, and compassion. I would maintain that, from a moral point of view, each member of society has a claim on the solicitude of all other members of the same society and a claim, according to need, on all of the resources of the same society. Only if we acknowledge such solicitude and the need, can we use the term "perspective," which envisions the widest possible deployment of resources for the widest enhancement of human life. How this deployment is to be brought about is the task of the citizens at large in a democratic but divided society.

NOTES

1. Aristotle, *Topics*, I, iv–v; 101b10–102b26.
2. Aristotle, *Metaphysics*, VII, vii; 1032a26.
3. Georges Buffon, *Histoire Naturelle et Particulaire* 1 (Paris: Impr. Royalle, 1770), 45ff.
4. Charles Darwin, *Origin of Species* (Cambridge, Massachusetts: Harvard University Press, 1964), 56.

5. Ibid., 51-52.

6. Ibid., 486-487.

7. F. Johann Gottfried Herder, *Ideas on the Philosophy of History*, tr. E. Quinet (London, 1827), vol 1, 346; vol 2, 3, 33-58.

8. Joseph de Maistre, *Considerations sur la France, Oeuvres* (1875), vol 1, 68.

ANNETTE DULA

Yes, There Are African-American Perspectives on Bioethics

African-Americans have a distinctive world view. Its diversity and power are reflected in our music from the blues of Bessie Smith, the gospel of Mahalia Jackson, and the jazz of Louie Armstrong to the rap of Run D.M.C. Our use of language, our hairstyles, our extended families, our religions, our art, our lifestyles—all testify to distinctive African-American world views. And, as we have perspectives and attitudes on health, sickness, death, and perspectives on life in general, so it follows that we have one on bioethics.[1]

PHILOSOPHICAL FOUNDATIONS

My purpose is to show you that there are good reasons to have an African-American perspective on bioethics. My talk is divided into three parts. First, I will argue that an African perspective on bioethics has foundations in health experiences and in a tradition of activist philosophy. Second, I will show through relevant examples that an unequal power relationship between white health care systems and their African-American clients has led to unethical medical behavior toward African-Americans in general. Third, I will argue that developing a professional perspective not only enriches the bioethical profession at large, but gives voice to the concerns of those not in the power circle and not able to speak for themselves.

Everyday I teach ethics to family practice residents in a clinical setting. One issue that recurs frequently is that of informed consent. Often people don't know what's being done to them; so I have made informed consent a second focus of my talk.

African-Americans have distinct world views or perspectives. These are responses to our experiences. Our history is one of unequal power relations, of oppression, domination, subordination, and ridicule. But as we have seen and heard, and despite our powerless status in this country, we have managed in many instances to respond creatively to such unfairness and to leave a distinctive, positive and indelible mark on Euro-American culture in the process.

Perspectives are based on class, race, and gender experiences. The experiences of poor people are different from those of rich people; those of African-Americans are different from those of Euro-Americans. Men and women's experiences differ. Rich people, white people and men have more power than African-Americans, poor people, or women. Thus, perspectives reflect power differentials or status in society.

THE HEALTH STATUS OF AFRICAN-AMERICANS

I suggest that our health status and our philosophy of life are two factors that shape an African-American bioethics. The first factor is our health status because health care and health levels reflect the general status of a group.

That there are great differences in the health of African-Americans and European-Americans is well documented. African-Americans receive less health care than Caucasians. More than twice as many African-Americans as whites are born with low birth weight.[2] Our babies die at almost twice the rate of white babies.[3] We do not live as long as whites do. For whites the average age span is 74 years; for African-Americans it is 69 years.[4] Self-reported data indicate that 50 percent more African-Americans than whites are likely to regard themselves in fair or poor health.[5] The mortality rate for heart disease in African-American males is twice that for white males. Recent research has shown that African-Americans tend to get less aggressive treatment for heart disease than do whites.[6] Cancer in whites is most likely to be localized; while in African-Americans, it is systemic. Therefore, more African-Americans than whites die from cancer, except for stomach cancer.[7]

African-Americans are included in fewer trials of new drugs.[8] Unfortunately, government programs do not target African-Americans as a group that needs special attention. If it did heed, African-American mortality and morbidity could be reduced by government-sponsored health programs. Research has shown that if African-Americans had the same death rate as other Americans, 59,000 African-American deaths a year would not occur.[9] Instead, government programs target general populations, such as the poor or pregnant women. Consequently, benefits to special populations are diffused. Clearly, the health status of African-Americans is a factor in shaping a distinctive African-American bioethics perspective.

Our unequal health situation is a result of three factors. Institutional racism has been an effective barrier to health care and, of course, has it roots in the historically unequal power relations between African-Americans and the medical profession and African-Americans and society at large.[10] It has worked effectively to keep African-American physicians out of the mainstream medical community, even though research has shown that a large percentage of African-American physicians return to minority communities to practice. Today, institutional racism in health care is manifested in the way African-Americans are treated and in the way that institutional views about poor people overlap with views about African-Americans. Both African-Americans and the poor experience long delays before they receive adequate health care, are unable to shop for services competitively, and often receive poor quality and discontinuous health care.

Economic inequality is another factor that contributes to our poor health. As DuBois said, "to be poor is hard, but to be a poor race in a land of dollars is the very bottom of hardships."[11] Our economic status reflects the kinds of jobs we have and the houses we inhabit—both of which can affect our health status. Poor people have poor health; and a disproportionate number of African-American people are poor. And lastly, it must be stated that the poor and African-Americans seek help later and not as often as middle-class people do.

Attitudinal and access barriers are yet a third factor in unequal health care. By attitudinal barriers, I mean our beliefs about the health care system, perceived racism, and our health values.[12] One recent study in *The Journal of the American Medical Association* revealed that African-Americans are less likely than white Americans to be satisfied with the way their physicians treat them, more dissatisfied with their hospital care, and more likely to believe that their hospital stay was too short.[13]

AFRICAN-AMERICAN ACTIVIST PHILOSOPHY

The second factor that could shape a distinctive perspective is African-American academic philosophy. The perspectives of many African-American philosophers differ from the perspectives of mainstream philosophers. Mainstream philosophers present philosophy primarily as a thinking enterprise. Analytical philosophy, as it is called, does not have a history of advocating for social change and transformation. With few exceptions, Euro-American philosophers have either gingerly approached or neglected altogether to comment on social ills and injustices such as slavery, racism, sexism, poverty, and class struggles.

In contrast, most African-American philosophers have always been concerned with social injustices. They view the world as members of an oppressed race, that is, through a cultural context of being the unequal partner in a relationship. Many African-American philosophers feel that academic philosophy devoid of social context is a luxury that African-American scholars can ill afford.[14]

African-American philosophers have purposely elected to use philosophy as a tool not only for naming, defining, and analyzing our social situation, but also for recommending, advocating, and sometimes harassing to achieve political and social empowerment—a stance contrary to Euro-American philosophical methods.[15]

Mainstream bioethics draws on mainstream philosophy; it cites Kant, Mill, Hume, and Nozick. An African-American bioethical perspective can and should draw on African-American philosophy. It should cite its own authorities: W.E.B. DuBois, Alain Locke, William Banner, Leonard Harris, Laurence Thomas, and others.

The concerns of bioethics and African-American philosophy overlap. Both are concerned, for example, with issues of distributive justice and fairness, with autonomy and paternalism in unequal relationships, and with addressing the ills of individuals and society. African-American philosophy is an appropriate source for bioethics in general and African-American bioethics in particular.

So far, I have argued that two factors shape our perspective. Our health care experiences are different from those of Euro-Americans. Our activist tradition in philosophy works to eliminate these differences. Thus, health care perspectives and African-American philosophy form a foundation for an African-American bioethics.

MAINSTREAM ISSUES RELEVANT TO AFRICAN-AMERICANS

I turn now to some more practical concerns. The history of unequal power relations explains abuses against African-Americans in the health care system. A look at this history reminds us of the sources of our perspectives. I suggest that mainstream bioethics issues have particular relevance for African-Americans. I will use two examples:

birth control and experimentation. These examples illustrate that we have concrete reasons to invest ourselves in the bioethics debate.

REPRODUCTIVE RIGHTS AND STERILIZATION

Issues centering around birth control and reproduction are central to many bioethical discussions today. Among these are family planning, sterilization, and genetic screening—questions of particular interest to African-American women because we have been exploited in each of these areas. Therefore, we may see these issues differently from white women. If we look at the history of birth control in North America, we can understand the source of one of these different perspectives.

The birth control movement in the United States is marked by three phases. The middle of the eighteenth century witnessed the beginning of the first phase of the birth control movement.[16] "Voluntary motherhood" was the rallying cry of the early feminists. Essentially, voluntary motherhood meant that women ought to be able to say no to their husbands as a means of limiting the number of children they bore. The irony of voluntary motherhood was that while white feminists were refusing their husbands' sexual demands, African-American women did not have the same right to say no to the husbands of those same early feminists. This is to say nothing of the fact that African-American women had been exploited as breeding wenches in order to produce a stock of slaves.

The second phase of the birth control movement actually gave rise to the phrase "birth control," which was coined by Margaret Sanger in 1915.[17] Initially, this stage of the movement led to the recognition that reproductive rights and political rights were intertwined. The practice of birth control would give white women the freedom to pursue new opportunities which their subsequent right to vote would soon make possible.[18] White women could go to work while African-American women cared for white children and did house work in white homes.

Unfortunately, the second stage of the birth control movement coincided with the eugenics movement in the first two decades of this century. When the white birth rate began to decline, eugenicists chastised middle-class white women for contributing to the suicide of the white race. As Paul Popenoe notes: "Continued limitation of offspring in the white race simply invites the black, brown, and yellow races to finish work already begun by birth control, and reduce the whites to a subject race."[19]

Eugenicists proposed two methods for curbing race suicide. On the one hand, middle-class white women had a moral obligation to have large families; on the other hand, poor immigrant women and African-American women had a moral obligation to restrict the size of their families because they were likely to be of inferior stock. On the basis of this argument, Guy Irving Burch of the American Eugenics Society advocated birth control for African-American and immigrant women. He notes: "We must prevent the American people from being replaced by alien or Negro stock, whether it be by immigration or by overly high birth rates among others in this country."[20] In addition, poor people created a drain on the taxes and charity of the wealthy.[21]

The woman's movement then adopted the ideals of the eugenicists regarding poor and minority women. Margaret Sanger saw the chief issue of birth control as "more children from the fit and less from the unfit."[22]

The 1940s marked the beginning of the third phase of birth control which was renamed, "Planned Parenthood."

In the 1950s, several states tried to extend sterilization laws to include compulsory sterilization of mothers of illegitimate children.[23] In the 1960s, the government began subsidizing family planning clinics. The purpose of these subsidies was to reduce the number of people on welfare by checking the transmission of poverty from generation to generation. The number of family planning clinics in an area was proportional to the number of African-Americans and Hispanics in the areas.[24] In Puerto Rico, by 1965, a third of the women had been sterilized.[25] In 1972 it was reported that there was a sevenfold rise in hysterectomies over the previous year at Los Angeles Hospital. These policies were influential in arousing African-American suspicions that there were racist motives behind family planning efforts.[26]

In 1973 two sisters, twelve-year-old Mary Alice Relf and fourteen-year-old Minnie Lee were surgically sterilized without consent. In the same town where they lived, eleven other young girls about the same ages as the Relf sisters had also been sterilized. Ten of these girls were African-American. In South Carolina, of thirty-four deliveries paid for by Medicaid, eighteen included sterilizations and all eighteen were young black women.[27] In 1972, Carl Schultz, Director of HEW's Population Affairs Office, estimated that between 100,000 and 200,000 sterilizations had been funded by the government.[28]

Thus, the first phase of the woman's movement completely ignored black women's sexual subjugation to white masters. And in the second phase, the movement adopted the racist policies of eugenics philosophy. The third stage saw a number of coercive measures supported by governmental policy to contain the population of African-Americans and poor people. While birth control per se was perceived as a benefit, African-Americans have historically objected to birth control as a method of dealing with poverty.

EXPERIMENTATION

Of course we cannot mention abuses without at least a minimal reference to the infamous Tuskegee experiment, which began in 1932 and continued until 1972, lasting forty years. Four hundred poor and poorly-educated syphilitic black men in Alabama were part of a government experiment to find out the course of untreated syphilis. The experiment was *sponsored* by the Public Health Service in 1932 and *condoned* by the Surgeon General in 1935. By 1936 the effects of nontreatment were already known. Still the experiment continued into the forties, fifties and sixties. In 1969, an ad hoc committee was appointed by the Public Health Service to review the Tuskegee study and the committee decided to continue it.[29]

In case you think that such things no longer occur, the April 1984 issue of *The American Journal of Public Health* reported that in the State of Maryland, 52,000 women were screened for sickle cell anemia and that of this number 13,000, or 38 percent, were screened without their consent.[30] These women were not given the benefit of prescreening education or follow-up counseling or the opportunity to decline screening. One wonders where the medical profession was.

One of the key ethical issues germane to unequal power relations is informed consent. In an unequal relationship informed consent may not be possible. The unequal partner may be forced to consent by powerlessness, poverty, coercion, or lack of understanding. Often, members of subordinate groups are not awarded full respect as persons, in which case their consent seems unnecessary.

I have shown that our experiences with health care suggest that we ought to take a particular interest in bioethics debates. We have also seen that abuse is likely to occur to powerless people, and that our perspective on bioethics derives from a history of being in an unequal power relationship. I have also shown that we do have a distinctive African-American perspective, based on our activist philosophy and our health care experiences. More than that, I have shown that the history of abuse that stems from the unequal power relationship commands our attention to bioethical issues. Now, in this third part of my paper, I argue that a professional perspective can give voice to the concerns of those not in the power circle. Let me present two examples where having a professional perspective has made a difference in social and political relations: African-American psychology and the woman's movement.

Until recently, psychology as a discipline viewed African-Americans as genetically and mentally inferior, incapable of abstract reasoning, culturally deprived, passive, ugly, lazy, childishly happy, dishonest, and emotionally immature or disturbed. Mainstream psychology owned these definitions and looked at African-Americans through a deficient model—a model that had been specifically constructed to explain African-American behavior.[31] This viewpoint became dominant not only in professional circles but also in the popular imagination and the media. When African-American psychologists gained entrance into the profession of psychology, they challenged that pathological model.[32] They presented an African-American perspective on psychology that addressed the ruling group's assessment of African-Americans and changed, to a certain extent, the way society looks at us.

The woman's movement is another example in which having a perspective makes a difference. Here I am speaking about the white woman's movement. Twenty years ago people were asking, "Should there be a woman's perspective on health?" This is no longer a question.

White women, like African-Americans, generally have a history of being oppressed and dominated; their perspective has been defined, for the most part, by men. Their voices, like African-American voices, have traditionally been unheard, ignored, or trivialized. Though the roots of the woman's movement in the United States go back to the 1850s, it was only in the foment of the civil rights movement in the 1960s and 1970s that tremendous gains were made. Women's voices were heard on a number of fronts: literature, psychology, and especially in health concerns. In the early seventies, emphasis was placed on reproductive rights. The unifying force of women was for "abortion on demand," culminating in Roe v. Wade. Some current issues include maternal and child health; the rights of women versus the rights of the fetus; unnecessary hysterectomies and caesareans, the doctor-patient relationship, and the empowerment of women. More recently, abortion rights have again assumed major importance in the woman's movement. Over the last couple of years, increasing numbers of women have also been drawn to the field of applied ethics, specifically to bioethics.[33]

In the development of African-American psychology and in the woman's movement, an articulated perspective has been effective in promoting pluralism. We still need to articulate our perspectives on

African-American bioethics and to join the mainstream debate so as to influence policy that affects African-Americans, poor and power-less people generally.

THE ANSWER IS YES

Yes, we do have an African-American perspective on bioethics. I have argued that we need to develop professional perspectives on bio-ethics to voice the concerns of African-Americans. These concerns fol-low from our experiences in society and in the health care system. As African-Americans, we have historically been the less powerful mem-bers of our society. Thus, it is our history and our experiences in un-equal power relationships that give us the right to develop distinctive bioethics perspectives.

There is a shocking history of medical abuse against powerless people. Often the form of the abuse is violation of informed consent. Indeed, the examples that I have presented share the two common el-ements of powerlessness and the absence of the informed consent. Consequently, I have suggested that in unequal relationships, in-formed consent does not work.

I use informed consent to show that there are issues in bioethics that are of particular reference to African-Americans. There is, how-ever, no lack of issues that require attention; I could just as easily have used surrogacy or abortion to demonstrate my point.

Broader questions of distributive justice are at stake. We are aware of the disturbing health differences between African-Ameri-cans and white Americans. As stated before, twice as many black ba-bies die as white babies. We should perhaps give special attention to this problem. For surely it is an ethical issue at least as important as a custody fight for frozen embryos.

Though there may be an acknowledged African-American per-spective on bioethics, that does not mean that our perspectives have been fully articulated. Rather we need to organize professionally to articulate our views further. That is the purpose of our symposium—to begin a process of identifying, developing, and establishing our positions as African-American bioethicists. This conference and its publications are an opportunity to hear and discuss our different per-spectives.

NOTES

1.   Herman J. Blake, "Doctor can't do me no good," in *Black Folk Medicine: The Therapeutic Significance of Faith and Trust*, ed. W. H. Watson (New Brunswick: Transaction Books, 1983).

2.   Antonia A. Rene, "Racial Differences in Mortality: Blacks and Whites," in *Health Care Issues in Black America*: Policies, Problems, and Prospects, ed. Woodrow Jones and Mitchell F. Rice (New York: Greenwood Press, 1987), 20-41.

3.   Dorothy C. Hanze, "Closing the Gap Between Black and White Infant Mortality Rates: An Analysis of Policy Options," in *Health Care Issues in Black America*, 119-139.

4.   *Report of the Secretary's Task Force on Black and Minority Health.* Department of Health and Human Services.

5.   Robert Blendon, Linda Arken, Howard Freeman, and Christopher Corey, "Access to Medical Care for Black and White Americans: A Matter of Continuing Concern," *The Journal of the American Medical Association*, 261 (1989): 278-281.

6.   Mark B. Wenneker and Arnold M. Epstein, "Racial Inequalities in the Use of Procedures for Patients with Ischemic Heart Disease in Massachusetts," *The Journal of the American Medical Association* 261 (1989): 253-257.

7.   Antonia Rene, "Racial Differences in Mortality," 20-41.

8.   Craig K. Svensson, "Representation of American Blacks in Clinical Trials of New Drugs," *The Journal of the American Medical Association* 261 (1989): 263-265.

9.   S. M. Miller, "Race in the Health of America," *The Milbank Quarterly* 65 (Supplement 2): 500-528.

10.   See *Health Care Issues in Black America*; also note 4 above.

11.   *The Souls of Black Folk: Essays and Sketches* (Greenwich, Connecticut: Faucett Publishing, Inc., 1961), 20.

12.   See note 10 above.

13.   Robert Blendon, et al. "Access to Medical Care," 278-281.

14.   Leonard Harris, *Philosophy Born of Struggle* (Dubuque: Kendall/Hunt, 1983).

15.   Ibid.

16.   Linda Gordon, *Woman's Body, Woman's Right: Birth Control in America* (New York: Penguin Books, 1976).

17.   Ibid.

18.   Angela Davis, *Women, Race and Class* (New York: Vintage Books, 1981).

19.   Paul Popenoe, *Conservation of the Family* (Baltimore: Williams and Wilkins, 1926), 144.

20.   Linda Gordon, *Woman's Body, Woman's Right*, 283.

21.   Ibid.

22.   Ibid., 281.

23.   Joseph L. Morrison, "Illegitimacy, Sterilization, and Racism: A North Carolina Case History," *Social Science Review* 39 (1965): 1-10.

24.   Ketayun H. Gould, "Black Women in Double Jeopardy: A Perspective on Birth Control," *National Association of Social Workers* (1984): 96-105.

25.   Bonnie Mass, *Population Target: The Political Economy. Population Control in Latin America* (Toronto: Women's Press, 1976).

26.   Davis, *Women, Race and Class.*

27.   Herbert Aptheker, "Racism and Human Experimentation," *Political Affairs* 53,2 (1974): 27-60.

28.   Les Payne, "Forced Sterilization for the Poor," *San Francisco Chronicle*, 26 Feb 1974.

29.   Herbert Aptheker, "Sterilization, Experimentation and Imperialism," *Political Affairs*, 53,2 (1974): 37-48.

30.   Mark R. Farfel and Neil A. Holtzmann, "Education, Consent and Counseling in Sickle Cell Screening Programs: Report of a Survey," *The American Journal of Public Health* 74 (1984): 373-375.

31.   Arthur Billingsley, *Black Families in White America*, (Englewood Cliffs: Prentice Hall, 1968); and Maxine Baca Zinn, "Family, Race and Poverty in the Eighties," *Signs* 14,4 (1989): 856-874.

32.   Adelbert H. Jenkins, *The Psychology of the Afro-American: A Humanistic Approach*, (New York, Pergamon Press, 1982).

33.   Morwenna Griffiths and Margaret Whitford, *Feminist Perspectives in Philosophy*, (Bloomington: Indiana University Press, 1988); Helen Bequaert Holmes, Betty B. Hoskins, and Michael Gross, ed. *Birth Control and Controlling Birth: Women Centered Perspectives* (Clifton, New Jersey, Humana Press, 1980).